DR SARAH BREWER trained ⬚⬚⬚⬚⬚⬚⬚⬚⬚⬚⬚ and gynaecology at Adde⬚⬚⬚⬚⬚⬚⬚⬚⬚ and has worked in gener⬚⬚⬚⬚⬚⬚⬚⬚⬚⬚⬚⬚⬚ clinics for many years. She ⬚⬚⬚ been a regular correspondent for the *Daily Mirror*, *The Daily Telegraph*, *Natural Health & Well-being*, *Prima* and *The Lady*. She was voted Health Journalist of the Year by the Health Food Manufacturer's Association in 2002. She is the author of over 40 popular health books including *The Encyclopedia of Vitamins, Minerals and Herbal Supplements*, and has a special interest in nutritional therapy.

Other titles in *The Daily Telegraph* series

The Daily Telegraph: Migraine
Valerie South

The Daily Telegraph: Sleep Really Well
Dr Paul Caldwell

The Daily Telegraph: Alzheimer's Disease
Dr William Malloy and Dr Paul Caldwell

The Daily Telegraph: Learning and Attention Disorders
Dr William Feldman

The Daily Telegraph: Chronic Pain
Arthur C. Klein

The Daily Telegraph: Backache
Sohel & Klein

The Daily Telegraph

MENOPAUSE
WHAT YOU REALLY NEED TO KNOW

DR SARAH BREWER

ROBINSON
London

Constable & Robinson Ltd
3 The Lanchesters
162 Fulham Palace Road
London W6 9ER
www.constablerobinson.com

First published in the UK by Robinson,
an imprint of Constable & Robinson Ltd, 2002

A copy of the British Library Cataloguing in Publication Data
is available from the British Library.

Publisher's Note: This book is not intended to be a substitute for
medical advice or treatment. Any person with a condition requiring
medical attention should consult a qualified medical practitioner
or suitable therapist.

ISBN 1-84119-662-2

Printed and bound in the EU

10 9 8 7 6 5 4 3 2 1

Contents

1
An Introduction to the Menopause

Are you reading this book because you dread the approach of the menopause? Perhaps you have watched a friend experience hot flushes and memory problems. Maybe you remember your mother's moods swinging wildly from irritability to anxiety. Perhaps you feel sad about this confirmation that you are no longer able to conceive a child and feel apprehensive about what the future holds. Despite some symptoms which can make you feel uncomfortable or unwell, the menopause is a natural event, not an illness. There is much you can do to ease your transition into this potentially rewarding time of life. Diet, exercise and stress management can all play an important role in helping you overcome physical and emotional problems. This book aims to tell you everything you need to know about the menopause so you can approach the change of life with confidence, knowing what to expect – and how to cope.

The menopause is often called the *change of life* although some call it the *climacteric*. The word *menopause* literally means the time when your last period stops. For most women, their last natural period occurs between the ages of 45 and 55, with a Western average of 51 years.

Although the menopause is dated from your last period, it is a process that starts five to ten years before, during your early to mid forties. This is the time when your level of the female hormone, oestrogen, naturally starts to fall. This loss of oestrogen is what triggers the menopause and is often accompanied by symptoms such as hot flushes and night sweats. As these symptoms start before the last period stops, and continue for some time afterwards, they are usually referred to as *perimenopausal* symptoms as they occur *around* the time of the menopause.

Every woman has a different experience of the menopause. Some quickly adapt to lower levels of oestrogen and notice few – if any – problems. Others find it harder and experience unpleasant symptoms that last from one to five years, occasionally longer. Lots of factors play a role in your response, including your diet, weight and lifestyle habits as well as the genes you have inherited. All these variables combine to affect the way your body adapts to lower levels of oestrogen. In general, if your hormone levels fall slowly, you will have fewer problems than if they suddenly plummet such as occurs after surgical removal of your ovaries.

Although the age at which your mother entered the menopause gives a good indication of when you can expect to have your menopause, the severity of symptoms will not necessarily be the same. Some doctors feel that expectations play a role, so that if you expect to suffer at the menopause, you are more likely to have a rough time. Even if your mother and sister had a terrible time, try not to assume the same thing will happen to you.

At least one in four women sail through with few problems, although three out of four suffer physical and emotional symptoms that can be troublesome. In particular, women who lead a demanding, stressful life seem more likely to suffer distressing symptoms. This is probably because their adrenal glands – which usually double their output of some sex hormones to make up for the lower levels produced by the ovaries – are already working flat-out at the menopause and do not have the reserves to produce increased amounts of hormones that can help to even out some of the fluctuations occurring around this time of life.

Although it is easy to pigeon-hole the menopause as a hormone deficiency disease, it is important to remember that it is a natural event. Your body is designed to stop making oestrogen and progesterone and to adjust to the changes this brings. Even so, the last thing most women want to bother with are distressing menopausal symptoms and long-term health problems linked with lowered levels of oestrogen.

Women are now in the best possible position to enjoy their postmenopausal years. On the one hand, hormone replacement therapy (HRT) – although controversial – is available for those who wish to use it short term. On the other, women can access a wide range of complementary therapies as well as making dietary and lifestyle changes to help ease them through what can – but doesn't have to be – a difficult time of life.

Many women choose to approach this phase of life in a natural manner. In some cultures, such as Japan for example, a high intake of dietary isoflavones (50 to 100 mg per day which is around thirty times higher than typical Western consumption) helps to reduce menopausal symptoms by improving oestrogen balance. As a result, less than 25 per cent of Japanese climacteric women complain of hot flushes, compared with 85 per cent of Western women.

Preparing for the Menopause

To help make your passage through the menopause easier, there are a number of steps you can take before your first symptoms start:

- try to eat a healthy diet, low in fat and containing plenty of fresh fruit, vegetables and unrefined, complex carbo-hydrates
- start increasing the amount of exercise you take to improve your fitness level
- try to lose any excess weight
- if you smoke, make a major effort to stop
- keep your alcohol limit to within the recommended safe maximum for women, of no more than two or three drinks per day, and try to have at least one alcohol-free day per week
- keep your stress levels as low as possible
- don't let yourself be over-burdened with tasks – learn to say 'no' and mean it, so that people don't put upon you
- find time for relaxation and quiet for at least half an hour per day – for example soaking in an aromatherapy bath surrounded with flickering candle-light is a great way to end the day.

This book will show you how you can approach and come through the menopause in the best way possible.

2
The Pre-menopausal Menstrual Cycle

The menopause marks the end of a woman's reproductive life, and occurs when the hormone cycle that synchronises changes in the ovaries and womb stops functioning. As this hormone cycle starts to wind down, many women find their periods become irregular, heavy or unusually light as the menopause approaches.

Regulation of the Menstrual Cycle

Before the menopause, the ovaries are regulated by two hormones, Follicle Stimulating Hormone (FSH) and Luteinising Hormone (LH), which are secreted in the pituitary gland at the base of the brain.

FSH triggers the production and development of several ovarian follicles (each containing an egg) at the start of each menstrual cycle. As well as growing in size, the developing follicles start to secrete the female hormone, oestrogen, and blood levels of oestrogen start to rise. One follicle usually starts to grow more rapidly than the others, and produces increasing amounts of oestrogen which feeds back onto the pituitary gland to damp down its production of FSH. As a result, blood levels of FSH fall slightly. When this happens, the other follicles stop growing, as only the dominant follicle has matured enough to continue responding to these lower FSH levels. As a result, only one egg is normally released each month. Contrary to popular belief, an egg is not released from alternate ovaries on alternate months. There doesn't seem to be a pattern and eggs are released from the two ovaries in an irregular and unpredictable pattern. Interestingly, egg cells seem to become less receptive in later life to the signals telling them to stop developing, so that two or more eggs may continue maturing and are released at ovulation. Women who conceive in their forties are therefore more likely to produce twins because of this super-ovulation phenomenon.

Just before ovulation, the pituitary gland releases a sudden surge of another menstrual regulatory hormone, Luteinising Hormone (LH), which acts as the signal to trigger ovulation 12–36 hours later. Once the egg has been released, the empty egg follicle collapses down to form a yellow cyst known as the corpus luteum. This yellow cyst secretes both oestrogen and progesterone, which together prevent other egg follicles developing for the remainder of the monthly cycle (this is the principle on which the combined oral contraceptive pill works) and also acts on the womb lining (endometrium) so it becomes more receptive to pregnancy should fertilization occur.

If fertilization does occur, the developing embryo secretes

a hormone, Human Chorionic Gonadotrophin (hCG), which prevents the corpus luteum from degenerating. The corpus luteum then continues secreting oestrogen and progesterone and maintains the early pregnancy by preventing menstruation. If pregnancy does not occur, however, the corpus luteum degenerates after about ten days. This causes a sharp fall in progesterone levels, which triggers the shedding of the outer womb lining as a period, and the start of a new menstrual cycle. In the meantime, the remains of the corpus luteum cyst are eventually replaced by scar tissue.

Normal Menstruation

The average age at which periods start (menarche) is 13.4 years, and the average age when they stop at the menopause is 51 years. From puberty until the menopause, women experience an average of 13 menstrual bleeds per year. Allowing for the lack of periods occurring during pregnancy, the average modern woman therefore experiences between 400 and 500 periods during her life. The menstrual fluid during a normal period varies between 30 ml and 75 ml. Therefore, throughout her life, a woman experiences a total menstrual fluid loss of between 13.5 and 33.75 litres (22.5–56.25 pints).

The length of the menstrual cycle varies, with anything between 21 and 35 days considered normal. For some women, however, the interval between periods may be 15 days or less, and in others 50 days or more – especially as the menopause approaches. The 28-day cycle quoted as the average only occurs in around 12 per cent of women.

Oestrogen and progesterone

Nearly all processes of female reproduction are regulated by the two female hormones, oestrogen and progesterone, acting together. They are both made in the female ovaries and enter the circulation, travelling round the body in the bloodstream until they recognize and interact with one of their special receptors on the wall of a body cell. The hormone then enters that cell and travels to the cell nucleus where it switches on certain genes. This triggers production of one or more proteins, including enzymes, to produce effects linked with either oestrogen or progesterone hormone.

Oestrogens

The ovaries produce several different female hormones that have a similar action and are together referred to as oestrogens. These include:

- oestradiol – the most potent form of oestrogen
- oestrone
- oestiol – the weakest oestrogen.

After producing their actions in the body, these three hormones are broken down in the liver to form a variety of weaker oestrogens. Some of these are excreted into the bile and squirted into the intestines, from where they are reabsorbed into the bloodstream. From the blood, unwanted oestrogen hormones are filtered out into the urine.

As well as helping to regulate the menstrual cycle, oestrogen has a number of other effects on your body. It can:

- stimulate growth of ovarian follicles
- stimulate growth of breasts
- increase production of new bone
- keep your tissues elastic – especially skin and blood vessel walls
- lower cholesterol levels and discourage hardening and furring up of the arteries
- increase blood flow to the uterus and growth of uterine muscle cells
- increase the motility of the fallopian tubes
- maintain female body shape and patterns of fat storage
- help to regulate your sex drive
- keep mucous membranes moist
- thin down skin oil secretions from sebaceous glands, making blackheads and spots less likely.

Progesterone

The word progesterone comes from the Latin *pro* and *gestatio* meaning *for pregnancy*. Progesterone is mainly secreted in the ovaries by cells surrounding the most fully developed egg, just before ovulation, and by the corpus luteum (yellow cyst) in the second half of the menstrual cycle. Blood levels of progesterone are highest during the third week of your menstrual cycle (days 21 to 23) then start to fall if fertilization has not occurred, and the corpus luteum fades away. If a fertilized egg does implant in the womb, however, it gives out a signal – human chorionic gonadotrophin – that keeps the corpus luteum going and progesterone levels increase.

Progesterone has several important effects in the female body. It:

- changes the growth phase of the womb lining to the secretory phase in preparation for receiving a fertilized egg
- maintains early pregnancy by preventing menstruation
- acts together with oestrogen to support production of breast milk
- relaxes smooth muscle cells in the uterus and elsewhere
- prevents production of Luteinising Hormone (LH) from the pituitary gland when progesterone levels are high – this prevents ovulation during pregnancy and to some extent during breast-feeding
- it changes cervical and vaginal mucus after ovulation, so that conception is less likely once a released egg has started to age
- has effects on salt and fluid retention which may be linked with pre-menstrual symptoms in some women.

Abnormal Menstruation Around the Menopause

As the menopause approaches, some women continue to have normal, regular periods, which just suddenly stop. It is more common to notice changes in your periods, however, and the menstrual pattern may become:

- irregular
- heavier than usual
- lighter than normal.

You should tell your doctor straight away if you notice:

- post-menopausal bleeding
- bleeding after intercourse

- unexpected bleeding (e.g. spotting) in between your periods.

Irregular Menstrual Bleeding

Irregular periods may come more frequently than normal (e.g. every 14 days or less) or less often (e.g. every two to three months). The commonest cause of an irregular cycle around the menopause is that ovulation fails to occur in some cycles. When ovulation fails, there is no empty follicle to develop into the corpus luteum and secrete progesterone hormone. Ovarian oestrogens continue to stimulate growth of your womb lining, however, which eventually becomes so thick it outgrows its blood supply. It then becomes starved of oxygen and starts to break down. The time taken for bleeding to occur is variable, but is usually less than 28 days from the onset of the previous period. Bleeding also varies from scanty to profuse. Other possible causes of irregular – especially infrequent – periods are:

- stress
- pregnancy
- being very overweight or significantly underweight
- over-active or underactive thyroid gland
- stopping the oral contraceptive Pill
- general illness
- polycystic ovaries (multiple small cysts on the ovaries)
- hormone imbalances.

Heavy Periods (Menorrhagia)

A heavy period can last for ten days or longer, with flooding and sometimes clots. One in ten women suffer from heavy periods at some time during their life, especially around the time of the menopause. As with irregular periods, a common cause is lack of ovulation, so the womb lining becomes excessively thick, leading to a period that is heavy as well as irregular. Other causes of heavy periods at this time of life include:

- fibroids (knot-like swellings in womb muscle)
- uterine polyps (fleshy growths in the womb lining)
- endometriosis (womb lining cells found outside the womb cavity)
- pelvic inflammatory disease (infection of the upper reproductive tract)
- rarely, cancer of the cervix, endometrium or ovary.

If you suffer from heavy periods, consult your doctor in case investigation and treatment are needed. If heavy bleeding is allowed to continue, it may lead to anaemia.

Although a progesterone-like hormone, norethisterone, is widely prescribed to reduce heavy bleeding, at most it reduces blood loss by 20 per cent and may even make bleeding worse. Other drug treatments are more successful – non-steroidal anti-inflammatory drugs such as mefenamic acid and naproxen can reduce blood loss by 20–45 per cent, while tranexamic acid (which stops blood clots redissolving) reduces blood loss by 45–60 per cent. Sometimes the contraceptive Pill may be suggested to reduce heavy periods, especially if you also need contraception. Another approach worth considering is the Mirena intra-uterine-system (a contraceptive coil that releases low doses of levonorgestrel hormone) which can reduce blood loss by 90 per cent after six months, although it may cause irregular bleeding initially.

Where drug treatment is ineffective, a hysterectomy may be advised as a final resort. Two-thirds of hysterectomies are carried out to treat heavy periods. Newer surgical options that remove just the womb lining (endometrium) using a laser, hot cutting wire or microwaves are becoming increasingly popular, and can be used in at least half of all women who would otherwise need a hysterectomy. After these techniques, around 40 per cent of women have no further periods, while another 40 per cent have a significantly reduced menstrual flow.

Painful Periods (Dysmenorrhoea)

The lining of the womb (endometrium) makes hormone-like chemicals called prostaglandins. These help the womb contract during a period to help ensure bleeding is not excessive. Some women suffer from excessive period pain, which usually starts with the onset of bleeding and lasts from several hours to several days. It tends to be spasmodic or colicky in nature and may be accompanied by diarrhoea, nausea and even vomiting. If pain is excessive, consult your doctor, as you may need investigation for problems such as fibroids or endometriosis.

Period pains seem to be significantly worse in women with a low intake of dietary fish oils, and taking omega-3 fish oil supplements has been shown to significantly improve painful periods. This is because they contain essential fatty acids that have a beneficial effect on the types of prostaglandins produced. Taking magnesium supplements has also been found to reduce back pain and lower abdominal pain associated with menstruation – especially on the second and third days – probably due to its muscle relaxant effect. Women who experience painful periods around the time of menopause may find these supplements helpful.

Pre-menstrual Syndrome (PMS)

Pre-menstrual syndrome is a common and distressing problem affecting as many as one in two women. It often becomes worse around the time of the menopause and may be prolonged when periods are missed or delayed. Usually, the symptoms of PMS start in the two weeks before a period is due and stop quickly once bleeding occurs. Even if your hormone levels are too low to trigger a period, as the menopause approaches, they can still cause symptoms of PMS.

Evening primrose oil contains hormone building blocks and will help to even out hormonal imbalances, but needs to be taken at doses of up to 3 g a day for at least three months before an effect may be noticed. It seems to be especially helpful in reducing low mood and cyclical breast pain. Vitamin B6 is helpful for fatigue and emotional symptoms such as depression and irritability, while magnesium supplements can reduce symptoms of irritability, depression, anxiety/tension, bloating, tiredness and headaches. Vitamin D and calcium appear to reduce headache, negative emotions, fluid retention and pain. Each supplement tends to help around two out of three women, but must be taken for at least three months to asses the effect. A recent randomized, placebo controlled trial of 170 women published in the *British Medical Journal* found that Agnus castus (see page 168) significantly reduced irritability, mood changes, headache and breast fullness.

Intermenstrual Bleeding

Bleeding between periods can take the form of spotting or a heavier loss, and may occur spontaneously or after making love. In many cases, no obvious cause is found although the possibility of a miscarriage or ectopic pregnancy needs to be explored.

A cervical erosion (more properly known as an ectropion) can cause bleeding between periods and occurs when delicate cells lining the cervical canal also cover an area on the outer cervix. This forms a red, velvety area that bleeds easily when touched. This is a normal result of oestrogen stimulation and is common in women on the Pill and during pregnancy. Sometimes, bleeding between periods is due to a cervical polyp, especially when bleeding occurs after sex. A polyp is a fragile, fleshy growth that can protrude through the cervical opening on a stalk. Infection and inflammation can also trigger vaginal bleeding and Chlamydia infection and pelvic inflammatory disease need to be ruled out.

If you using a hormonal method of contraception (e.g. oral contraceptive pill, mini pill, Depot injection or Mirena intra-uterine system) you could be experiencing breakthrough bleeding and your doctor can advise whether or not you need to use an additional method of contraception to prevent an unplanned pregnancy until other causes have been ruled out.

Occasionally, bleeding between periods or after sex is due to cancer of the cervix, womb or ovary, although this is uncommon. Another possible cause of bleeding between periods is a hormone imbalance.

Any woman who notices any bleeding between periods should always seek medical advice, even if it is only slight spotting.

Post-Menopausal Bleeding

Most women breathe a sigh of relief when the menopause approaches and their periods stop, especially where they have suffered from painful periods and/or pre-menstrual syndrome. Any vaginal bleeding appearing more than six months after you thought your periods had stopped should not be dismissed as just one of those things, however, but should always be taken seriously, even if it's only a little spotting. In nine out of ten cases, nothing abnormal is found, so try not to panic. However, one per cent of single episodes of post menopausal bleeding and 10 per cent of recurrent episodes of post menopausal bleeding may be due to a gynaecological cancer. If diagnosed early, your chance of successful treatment is greatly improved.

One of the commonest causes of post menopausal bleeding is a doctor prescribing HRT and forgetting to warn the woman that her monthly period may return. Other causes include:

- thinning of vaginal tissues due to lack of oestrogen
- trauma during intercourse, especially after a time of sexual abstinence
- a polyp on the cervix or endometrium
- fibroids
- over-stimulation of the endometrium (cystic hyperplasia) due to excessive doses of oestrogen (e.g. where oestrogen HRT, but no progestogen is taken by a woman who has not had a hysterectomy).

Menstrual Chart

If your periods are causing problems around the menopause, it is worth keeping a menstrual diary like the one below which you can show to your doctor. This will help you keep track of when you bleed or have troublesome symptoms. Start the first month on the first day of your period (day 1) and start a new line with each period. Use different symbols for different events.

Days Of Cycle

	1 2 3 4 5 6 7 8 9 10 11 12 13 14 15 16 17 18 19 20 21 22 23 24 25 26 27 28 29 30
Month 1	XX ! ! ! ! ! X H H H H H H D I DI HBD B B o o – –
Month 2	
Month 3	

Symbols – use your own examples

o = Spotting   X = Light bleeding   ! = Heavy bleeding   H = Hot Flushes

D = Depression   I = Irritability   P = Pain   T = Tiredness   B = Bloating

Understanding your menstrual cycle is a key early step in helping you assess the effects of the onset of menopause.

3
The Onset of Menopause

At birth, a baby girl is born with ovaries that contain a full complement of around 2 million immature eggs (oocytes). Unlike a male, who only starts producing sex cells (sperm) at puberty and continues churning them out until the end of his days, she will never produce any more eggs throughout her life. On the contrary, she will rapidly start to lose them. Many immature eggs disintegrate and are reabsorbed during childhood so that, by the time of puberty, only a quarter of these eggs remain – around half a million – to last until the menopause.

What Triggers The Menopause?

The menopause is triggered as the ovaries run out of eggs. While you had around half a million eggs at the time of puberty, these disappear or stop responding to hormone signals at an average rate of around 1,000–1,500 per month.

On top of this, around 15 eggs start to develop and mature during each monthly cycle, although only one is usually released at ovulation each month. At some stage during the age range 45–55, your supply of eggs will have dwindled to the extent that an irregular number start developing each month.

Oestrogen hormone is mainly produced by a cluster of cells surrounding each egg which together form an ovarian follicle. As the ovaries start to run out of eggs, and the follicles that remain start to age, disintegrate or stop responding to hormone signals, your oestrogen levels also start to fall – purely because not enough egg follicles remain to make all the oestrogen you need. The pituitary gland in the brain senses this and tries to kick-start your tiring ovaries by increasing its secretion of Follicle Stimulating Hormone (FSH) and Luteinising Hormone (LH). Both of these are thought to contribute to menopausal symptoms such as hot flushes and night sweats.

As your oestrogen levels fall, the womb lining loses its main source of stimulation. In many cases, while your ovaries produce enough oestrogen to stimulate growth of your womb lining, it is not enough to trigger ovulation. As a result, your periods will become irregular, and may be unusually heavy or unusually light. Your periods will eventually stop when the ovaries have only a few thousand eggs remaining which cannot secrete enough oestrogen to keep the menstrual cycle ticking over.

For most women, the age at which her mother reaches the menopause is a good guide to when she will go through it herself. A few other factors also determine when your menopause will occur: – for example smoking cigarettes, stress and having a hysterectomy even though your ovaries are left behind.

Premature Menopause

As many as one in ten women may enter the menopause before the age of 45. When the last natural period occurs before the age of 40, however, it is classed as premature and known medically as premature ovarian failure. A natural premature menopause affects an estimated 1–2 per cent of women, with a further 8 per cent of women experiencing an early menopause as a result of medical or surgical treatment. Going through an early menopause can be a devastating experience, especially if you were hoping for a future pregnancy. It can threaten your sexuality and self-esteem and make you feel angry, cheated, isolated or old before your time. If a woman who has experienced a premature menopause wishes to have a baby, she will need to undergo assisted fertility techniques using eggs donated by another woman.

If you find yourself in an emotional turmoil as a result of an early menopause, it is important to seek help. Your GP can refer you to a counsellor and to a gynaecologist who specializes in the problems linked with early menopause.

Often the cause of an early menopause remains unknown, although a number of factors can play a role. It may be triggered when the immune system for some reason starts to make antibodies aimed against the ovaries – in effect, the body is attacking part of itself. In other women there is a genetic link – they may have inherited fewer egg follicles than normal, or eggs with a shorter lifespan. Recent research confirms that if your mother had her last period before the age of 45 years, you are more likely to as well. The study compared 22 pairs of identical twins, 37 pairs of non-identical twins, and 243 non-twin sisters, and estimated that, for non-twin sisters, age at menopause was 85–87 per cent due to genetic factors (70–71 per cent for twins). As you don't know which genes you have inherited, however, menopausal ages between relatives are still difficult to predict.

Heavy Smoking

The more you smoke, the sooner your periods tend to cease – heavy smokers can reach the menopause 18–24 months earlier than non-smokers. Several chemicals found in cigarette smoke (e.g. nicotine, arabinase, conitine) interfere with enzymes that process oestrogen hormone, so smoking both reduces the amount of oestrogen produced and increases the rate at which it is broken down.

Stress

Psychological factors can affect the menstrual cycle – when a woman is under stress, for example, she may miss a period. Similarly, it seems that stress can in some cases trigger the menopause, although this is poorly understood. It can certainly cause symptoms that are worse than in women who are not experiencing excess stress (see pages 219–228). Traumatic events such as illness, severe financial problems, or the death of a close relative can all be followed by a sudden stopping of periods.

Alcohol Intake

Excessive alcohol intake can lower oestrogen levels, shrink the ovaries and trigger a premature menopause. The intake that causes these problems varies from person to person, depending on how your metabolism handles alcohol and how much exercise you take. Guidelines suggest that women should drink no more than two or three units of alcohol per day, with at least one or two alcohol-free days per week. Weekly intakes of over 35 units are considered dangerous for women.

Infection

Infection with the mumps virus can cause inflammation of the ovaries and damage large numbers of egg follicles. This is rare, but may result in an early menopause.

Are you likely to have early menopausal symptoms?

- Does an early menopause run in your family?
- Do you smoke 20 cigarettes a day, or more?
- Have you had a hysterectomy?
- Do you regularly drink more than 35 units of alcohol per week?
- Have you started developing irregular periods, hot flushes or other menopausal symptoms before the age of 40?

Medical Treatments

Some types of drug treatment may temporarily or permanently affect the ovaries to produce symptoms of an early menopause.

Danazol Treatment with danazol for example, triggers a reversible, temporary menopause. It is a synthetic form of the male hormone, testosterone, and is used to treat a number of gynaecological conditions, including endometriosis, fibrocystic breast disease, heavy periods (menorrhagia) and pre-menstrual syndrome.

Danazol works directly on the ovaries to interfere with the enzymes responsible for the production of oestrogen and progesterone, and also affects the hypothalamus in the brain to lower secretion of gonadotrophin releasing hormone (GnRH – see below). This results in lowered oestrogen levels – similar to those found after the menopause – and danazol is therefore classed as a reversible, pseudomenopausal (false menopause) drug. While taking it, the ovaries stop making oestrogen and eggs stop ripening.

Three out of four women taking danazol will notice several body changes, of which many mimic the symptoms of the menopause (for example, hot flushes), while others are due to changing from a female hormone environment to a more masculine one (for example, muscle development and excess body hair). Once danazol is stopped, periods usually return to normal within three to eight weeks and the false menopause symptoms disappear.

GnRH Analogues A group of drugs called the GnRH analogues (buserelin, goserelin, leuprorelin, nafarelin, triptorelin) produce a reversible, false menopause and are used to treat gynaecological conditions such as endometriosis and breast cancer. The drugs work by interfering with production of gonadotrophin releasing hormone (GnRH) in the hypothalamus of the brain. GnRH is what triggers secretion of Follicle Stimulating Hormone (FSH) and Lutenising Hormone (LH) from the pituitary gland and these two hormones in turn act on the ovary to stimulate production of oestrogen and progesterone.

GnRH analogues bind to the pituitary gland at the sites (receptors) where GnRH usually triggers its action. But instead of quickly dropping off to free up the receptor again, as natural GnRH does, the drug sits on its receptors for several hours. When the drug first binds to the receptors, it stimulates production of FSH and LH, but as it continues to sit there, the pituitary gland becomes over-stimulated and drained so that it stops making both FSH and LH. Levels of FSH and LH start to go up for three to ten days before starting to go down again, and a reversible, false menopause is usually triggered after about two weeks.

Because they produce a false menopause, GnRH analogues can trigger a range of menopausal symptoms. They are so effective in producing an artificial menopause that they can also produce long-term effects of thinning bones (osteoporosis) and increased risk of heart attack. Treatment with GnRH analogues is therefore usually restricted to a single course of no longer than 6 months, except in special circumstances.

One possible solution is to replace some oestrogen or progesterone to prevent this happening, or to combine a small dose of danazol with the GnRH analogue, as danazol helps to increase bone density slightly.

Most women restart their periods within six to eight weeks of stopping treatment. Rarely, a woman using a GnRH analogue may enter the menopause while on treatment and not restart her periods once therapy stops.

Anti-oestrogen Drugs A group of drugs that block the action of oestrogen are used to treat some hormone-responsive gynaecological conditions such as breast cancer (e.g. tamoxifen, toremifene). When given to pre-menopausal women, they sometimes produce a reversible loss of periods (amenorrhoea) and menopause-like symptoms such as hot flushes. A newer class of drug, known as non-steroidal aromatase inhibitors (e.g. anastrozole, letrozole) block the conversion of androgens (male hormones) to oestrogens in peripheral tissues, such as body fat stores, and are also used to treat advanced breast cancer in post-menopausal women in whom anti-oestrogen therapy has failed. As these drugs lower oestrogen levels even further, they can also cause menopausal symptoms such as hot flushes, sweating and vaginal dryness.

Chemotherapy Drugs Chemotherapy and/or radiotherapy to treat cancer can temporarily, or permanently, affect the ovaries and may trigger an early menopause. Younger women have a better chance of their ovaries recovering than older women, but this will usually depend on the type of treatment given and the risk should be fully discussed with the woman before she decides whether or not to go ahead. It is usually possible for a section of ovarian tissue, complete with egg follicles, to be removed and frozen before treatment. This gives the woman a chance of having fertility treatment using her own eggs in the future.

Surgical Treatment Hysterectomy before the age of 40 will cause an early menopause if your ovaries are removed at the same time.

Different surgeons have different approaches to removing or conserving the ovaries during hysterectomy. The disadvantage of having the ovaries out is that you will have an instant, surgically induced menopause which usually produces severe symptoms unless HRT is started quickly. The advantage of having your ovaries removed – especially as the menopause approaches – is that you will never develop ovarian cancer. This is an important point, as it is estimated that one in 500 women whose ovaries are left inside will eventually develop an ovarian malignancy. Even where your ovaries are left intact:

- one in four women develop menopausal symptoms within two years
- on average, you will go through the menopause four years earlier – around the age of 47 – than a woman who has not had a hysterectomy.

The most likely reason is that the operation reduces ovarian blood supply. Alternatively, there may be some as-yet unrecognized interaction between the ovaries and uterus that causes the ovaries to fail more quickly once a hysterectomy is performed.

Resistant Ovaries

Some women experiencing a premature menopause have not run out of eggs, but those that are present have stopped responding to the normal hormone cycle. This is known as resistant ovary syndrome. In some cases the ovaries may recover spontaneously. The only way to diagnose this is through a biopsy to see if living egg follicles are present in ovarian tissue.

Complications of Premature Menopause

Because loss of oestrogen is one of the main causes of bone thinning, women experiencing an early menopause are at increased risk of osteoporosis. As oestrogen helps to protect against hardening and furring up of the arteries, you will also have a higher risk of high blood pressure, coronary heart disease and stroke than if your periods continued for longer (see Chapter 6). On the positive side, women who experience an early menopause are at less risk of some hormone-dependent problems such as fibroids and breast cancer.

Signs the Menopause is Approaching

For some women, the first sign that they have reached the menopause is when their perfectly normal, regular periods suddenly stop. This is unusual, however. Most women notice their periods changing and becoming irregular, lighter or heavier than usual and other early symptoms. If you experience problems with your periods, it is important to consult your doctor for advice – especially if you experience heavy bleeding.

Other early symptoms of the menopause can include:

- hot flushes and night sweats
- difficulty sleeping
- anxiety, irritability or mood swings that appear out of the blue
- unusual tiredness
- vaginal dryness
- headaches
- pins and needles
- poor concentration
- feelings of distance from those around you
- sudden difficulty coping with things you previously took in your stride.

If your doctor is unsure whether or not your symptoms are due to an approaching menopause, a blood test can help make the diagnosis.

Tests and Investigations to Confirm the Menopause

A blood test to measure levels of FSH and LH from the pituitary gland can show whether or not you are approaching the menopause.

FSH and LH are produced by the pituitary gland to stimulate egg and hormone production in the ovaries. Levels of FSH and LH usually peak in the middle of your cycle, just before ovulation occurs. As your ovaries produce less and less oestrogen as the menopause approaches, your pituitary gland increases its output of FSH and LH in an attempt to boost ovarian action. When FSH and LH reach a certain level, they are said to be in the 'menopausal range', as the ovary is obviously no longer responding to its usual signals. The following blood levels taken together are usually diagnostic of the menopause:

- an FSH level above 25 U/l
- an LH level above 50 U/l and
- an oestradiol (oestrogen) level of less than 150 pmol/l.

Occasionally, some women with FSH and LH levels in the menopausal range will return to a normal menstrual cycle if the ovaries suddenly start responding to FSH and LH again. This is not common, but a woman cannot assume that she is no longer fertile, as pregnancy can sometimes occur during the year or two after the last menstrual period, so you still need to use an effective method of contraception (see Chapter 14).

Menopausal Symptoms/Effects

The menopause can produce a number of symptoms, or effects, as your body adapts to lower oestrogen and progesterone levels, as follows.

Short-Term Effects starting during the perimenopause and lasting two to five years on average:

- hot flushes
- night sweats
- difficulty sleeping
- headaches
- tiredness
- anxiety
- irritability
- mood swings
- vaginal discomfort
- urinary problems
- poor memory
- poor concentration.

If you are using the combined, oral contraceptive Pill, the hormones it contains will mask these early symptoms of the menopause. If you are a non-smoker and your doctor has agreed that you can continue using this method of contraception right up until the menopause, you may not realise you have reached the change of life until you stop taking the Pill and your periods fail to return.

Medium-term Effects usually start after your last period, but may develop before and can last indefinitely:

- vaginal dryness
- painful intercourse
- loss of sex drive
- urinary symptoms
- thinning skin
- joint aches and pains
- urinary stress incontinence.

Long-term Effects starting anytime after the last period, but not usually for at least 5 years, worsening with time:

- heart disease
- osteoporosis.

The following chapters examine in more detail the nature of these symptoms and their implications.

4
Short-term Effects

In the five to ten years leading up to the menopause itself, your body starts going through a variety of changes. As oestrogen levels fall, tissues that are responsive to the hormone lose an important source of stimulation. These tissues include the:

- vagina and surrounding areas (vulva)
- uterus
- breasts
- bones
- heart and blood vessels
- brain
- urethra and bladder
- skin and mucous membranes
- hair follicles.

The most common short-term physical, emotional and psychological symptoms are hot flushes (75 per cent of women), night sweats (40 per cent), tiredness (40 per cent), irritability (30 per cent), mood swings (30 per cent), insomnia (30 per cent), vaginal discomfort (30 per cent), urinary problems (30 per cent) and depression (30 per cent).

These symptoms can begin before, during or after the time of the last natural period and usually last for up to two to five years, although they can go on for longer. The rate at which your oestrogen levels fall helps to determine how bad your symptoms are. If your oestrogen levels fall off relatively slowly, your body is designed to cope with what is a normal biological event, so that you do not suffer unduly. If your hormone levels fall quickly, however, your body has little time to adapt and you are plunged into the deep end of the changes occurring as a result of oestrogen withdrawal.

Overall, around a quarter of women sail through the menopause with few immediate problems except a few hot flushes that settle quickly. Around half of women class their symptoms as mild to moderate, while a further quarter feel they suffer more than expected.

Symptoms seem to be worse if you have been under prolonged stress. Usually, up to 5 per cent of circulating sex hormones are made by the adrenal glands. As your ovaries stop working, the adrenal glands take over some of their function and produce small amounts of oestrogen as well as doubling their output of testosterone-like male hormones (androgens). Some of these androgens have a weak oestrogen-like action or can be converted into oestrogens by other tissues in your body, especially your stores of fat.

If you have been under long-term stress, however, your adrenal glands may already be working flat out producing stress hormones such as adrenaline. As a result, when the menopause approaches, they have no extra reserves to boost their output of sex hormones. Stressed women therefore tend to suffer more and worse menopausal symptoms than women who are more in control of their life. They are also more likely to lose their sex drive. For advice on coping with stress, see page 219.

Short-term Physical Symptoms

These tend to start before your periods end. One in ten women get over them within six months, although one in 20 women experience menopausal symptoms off and on for ten years or more. Usually, your body finds a new balance at a lower level of oestrogen hormone, so symptoms become less troublesome.

Hot Flushes

Hot flushes are the most common menopausal symptom. They often first appear quite early on in the perimenopausal period, before you notice significant changes in your periods. In some women, they occur only over a short time, coinciding with a larger than usual fluctuation in hormone levels. In most cases, the tendency towards hot flushes passes within one or two years, although it may last for five years or more.

Each hot flush usually last from one to five minutes, although occasionally one may last an hour or more. Some women suffer at least one per day, while others may only get one per week. A few unlucky women seem to get several per hour – some claim to suffer as many as 50 hot flushes in a day – but it is unusual to have them this badly. Few women suffer more than 12 hot flushes per day.

The flush is usually felt over the upper trunk, neck, face and arms. Blood vessels in the skin dilate to increase blood flow so that your skin becomes red and hot. Skin temperature rises by 1–4 degrees Celsius, enough to make you feel sweaty and uncomfortable, although your internal body temperature stays much the same. By opening up blood vessels in your skin, your heart has to work harder to pump blood around your circulation, so your pulse rate usually goes up. Many women also have a premonition that the flush is on its way, and may feel unusually anxious, unwell, or notice sensations of skin tingling, prickling, pins and needles or pressure in their head. Others may feel dizzy and light-headed as their blood vessels dilate and blood pressure goes down.

Hot flushes are the body's way of trying to lose excessive heat. Flushing causes dilation of veins near the surface of the skin, so heat radiates off you. Sweating uses excessive heat to help sweat evaporate off the skin. An increased breathing rate means you literally blow off some heat through your lungs, while loss of appetite may occur to slow production of heat during digestion. Similarly, you may feel sluggish, which is the body's way of slow production of heat during physical activity.

Hot flushes can be triggered by a number of factors, including:

- hot surroundings
- increased humidity
- alcohol
- caffeine
- hot food or hot drinks
- spicy foods
- exposure to cigarette smoke
- strong emotions
- stress

- tiredness
- some drugs.

Try to identify any triggers you may have and avoid them as much as possible. One of the worst things about a hot flush is that it is such a visible sign that you are suffering a menopausal problem. Unfortunately, worrying about having a flush in public is likely to bring one on and to make it worse.

Researchers are still unsure of the exact cause of a hot flush. It was thought to be linked with increased levels of FSH and LH, as just before a flush there seems to be a surge of activity in the hypothalamus. This releases a master hormone known as GnRH, although no definite link between hormone levels and hot flushes has been found.

The most popular current theory is that hot flushes are due to changes in the metabolism of a brain chemical (noradrenaline) produced by falling levels of oestrogen. This affects the setting of the body's thermostat, which is regulated in the hypothalamus in the brain – next door to where GnRH is produced. Noradrenaline is also affected by stress, which is probably why stress can trigger a hot flush.

The body's responses to excessive heat or cold are regulated by different parts of the hypothalamus:

- stimulation of the front (anterior) part of the hypothalamus causes flushing and sweating and in extreme cases can reset the body's thermostat from 37 degrees to as much as 43 degrees (e.g. during a fever)
- stimulation of the back (posterior) part of the hypothalamus produces shivering.

Special cells making GnRH are sandwiched between these two areas. For some reason, the temperature regulation system does not work very well when oestrogen levels are lower than normal. It may be that as cells in the hypothalamus make more and more GnRH to trigger release of FSH and LH from the pituitary gland in an attempt to kick-start the failing ovaries (see page 23), the nearby temperature regulation system is over-stimulated.

Women who suffer from hot flushes seem to be more sensitive to lowered oestrogen levels than women who do not flush and tend to develop more – and worse – menopausal symptoms than those who do not flush.

If you develop a flush, don't be embarrassed. Breathe in deeply, sit still and try to relax.

Combating a hot flush

- Concentrate on breathing deeply and slowly
- Cool down with a chilled drink, sucking an ice-cube or eating ice cream
- Try to sit down near an open window or door so you can breathe fresh, cool air
- Carry a small, battery-operated personal fan in your bag for emergencies
- Carry a small packet of wet wipes to help you freshen up until you can wash or change
- Carry a small wash bag around with you containing flannel, soap, towel and deodorant plus a crease-proof change of clothes, if necessary.

Some women even enjoy their hot flushes, and find them useful – especially in winter when they have previously been sensitive to the cold.

Night Sweats

A hot flush is often followed by profuse sweating, especially at night – hence the name. You may find you wake drenched and with an unpleasant sensation of difficulty breathing, or you may wake feeling cold and clammy. You may be so drenched in sweat that you need to change your nightie and bed linen. Some women suffer from cold sweats rather than hot sweats and feel clammy and chilled. More usually, feelings of hot and cold alternate. As the body heats up, sweating occurs to cool you down again and is often so successful that you soon start shivering and pulling the covers back over yourself.

Researchers are unsure why bad hot flushes and sweats seem to occur at night. The activity of your hypothalamus and pituitary gland seems to peak at night between 1 a.m. and 3 a.m., but there is no proven link between your hormone levels and the occurrence of night sweats. If you are awoken at night with a sweat or flush, you may be one of the lucky ones who are able to freshen up then go straight back to sleep. More usually, you will lie there tossing and turning and find sleep difficult, or briefly sleep before waking up again every half hour.

If you fall into the sleep difficulty pattern, you are likely to become deficient in REM (rapid eye movement) sleep and end up feeling exhausted during the day. It can also lead to depression. Hormone replacement therapy has been shown to increase the time a woman spends in REM sleep. See pages 233–4 for self help tips on how to sleep better.

Dealing with night sweats

One of the most useful aids for a night sweat is to have a small office fan by the side of your bed – flinging off the bed clothes and switching on a cool breeze will soon make you feel more comfortable. Keeping a bottle of chilled mineral water in the bedroom (e.g. in a wine cooler) will also help you to freshen up as you sip it slowly.

- Try using sheets and layers of blankets rather than a duvet, so you can quickly adjust the amount of covers on your side of the bed
- Keep spare sheets easily to hand for a quick change when the bed is drenched – there's nothing worse than trying to get back to sleep in a wet bed
- Sleep with several single sheets and two duvets on a double bed, so you disturb your sleeping partner less.

Difficulty Sleeping

Even if you don't have sleep problems due to hot flushes or night sweats, you may develop insomnia due to oestrogen withdrawal.

Sleep is a form of unconsciousness which is your natural state of rest. This is essential for physical and mental well-being as it is a time of rest, rejuvenation and regeneration. Growth hormone is secreted in increased amounts during sleep, muscles and joints recover from constant use during the day, and most of the body's repair work is carried out – more skin, red blood cells, immune cells, intestinal lining cells and hair follicle cells are produced during sleep than when you are awake. Protein in all parts of the body is replenished faster during sleep as well, yet there is no con-clusive evidence that sleep is essential for any body organ except the brain. Even here, researchers are stumped as, para-doxically, the brain is actually more active during sleep than when you are wide awake.

The brain contains oestrogen receptors, and the

menopause does affect your natural sleep pattern. There are two main types of sleep:

- Rapid Eye Movement (REM) sleep in which the eyes are constantly on the move.
- Slow Wave (or non-REM sleep) in which the eyes are relatively still.

There are four stages of Slow Wave sleep – the lightest is Stage 1 and the deepest, Stage 4. When you first fall asleep, you rapidly pass through stages 1 and 2, then spend 70–100 minutes in stages 3 and 4. Sleep then lightens and a short period of around ten minutes REM sleep follows. This cycle repeats four to six times throughout the night, but as morning approaches, more and more time – up to one hour – is spent in REM sleep.

Interestingly, people who sleep only five hours per night tend to get a similar amount of slow wave sleep as those who regularly sleep eight hours per night – additional time spent sleeping is spent in REM sleep.

On average, you spend the following amount of time in each stage of sleep:

- Stage 1   5 per cent of the night (light sleep)
- Stage 2   50 per cent
- Stage 3   5 per cent
- Stage 4   15 per cent (deep sleep)
- REM   25 per cent.

Your sleep pattern naturally changes throughout life. As you get older, you spend less and less time in Stage 4 (really deep) sleep, so that by the age of 70, most people get no Stage 4 sleep at all. As sleep tends to be light, it is common for older people to wake several times during the night, though they may not recall this next morning.

Researchers have recently found that low oestrogen levels are linked with having less REM sleep, although the women affected are not necessarily sleep deprived. Sleep problems are usually helped by hormone replacement therapy, which also improves your sleep structure, increasing the amount of time you spend in REM sleep.

Other common sleep problems around the time of the menopause include difficulty going off to sleep or waking early in the morning. Early morning waking is one of the biological symptoms of depression, so if you also feel low in mood and burst into tears easily, it is important to seek help.

Vaginal Dryness

Vaginal dryness usually comes on a year or more after you first develop other menopausal symptoms such as hot flushes. Over half of all women develop vaginal dryness after the menopause that is bad enough to need treatment. This is because oestrogen is needed to switch on secretion of vaginal lubrication. Sex may become uncomfortable or painful and may even result in bleeding from thinning tissues. Most women notice some difficulties with intercourse, including loss of sex drive. Eventually, vaginal tissues – including the clitoris – will shrink, which can have a devastating effect on your sex life. Women who develop lack of lubrication can often be helped by the advice to use a water-based lubricant before making love (See Chapter 14). Using local oestrogen creams/gels or taking HRT will reverse and overcome these changes.

A natural form of vaginal oestrogen replacement is now

also available in the form of an isoflavone gel (called PhytoSoya), which contains plant-based oestrogen-like hormones that also supply useful lubrication.

Bladder Problems

The tissues of the bladder and urethra (tube through which urine flows from the bladder to the outside world) are also sensitive to oestrogen withdrawal. As a result, many menopausal women develop symptoms such as:

- wanting to go to the loo more often than usual (frequency)
- having to rush to the loo to pass urine (urgency)
- only passing small amounts of urine
- leaking of urine (stress incontinence)
- increased risk of bladder infection (cystitis).

Most of these problems can be overcome with pelvic floor exercises, hormone replacement therapy (local or systemic) or diet and lifestyle changes.

As the bladder symptoms of oestrogen withdrawal are similar to those of infection (cystitis), it can be difficult to know which is causing your problem. In general, if passing urine stings or burns, if your urine smells unpleasant, or if you notice blood in your urine, an infective cystitis is likely. (If in doubt, always seek medical advice and take a sample of urine along to the surgery with you. This can be tested for signs of bacterial infection (e.g. pus cells, presence of chemicals called nitrites.)

Menopausal Migraine

Migraine is common enough to affect one in ten people.

Attacks usually begin around puberty, then strike intermittently until middle age. Three quarters of all sufferers are aged between 16 and 45. For some sufferers, however, symptoms continue into older life.

As oestrogen has such a profound effect on blood vessels throughout your body – especially small ones – migraine is three times more common in women than men. Lots of women find they develop migraine for the first time during the menopause, which then improves as oestrogen-withdrawal symptoms fade away.

Migraine is usually only felt on one side of the head or is worse on one side (unilateral). It often centres around one eye and is accompanied by abdominal and/or visual symptoms. In contrast, a tension headache is a severe, continuous pressure felt on both sides of the head (bilateral). It can be felt over the top of the skull (vertex), over the back of the head (occiput) or above both eyes. It may feel like a tight, constricting band, or a non-specific ache. Tension headaches can occur at any age, but are also more common around the time of the menopause. They are linked with stress and depression.

There are two main sorts of migraine:

- *migraine without aura* or common migraine, consists of a severe, throbbing, pulsating or hammering headache on one side, usually with abdominal symptoms. These include loss of appetite, nausea, vomiting, dislike of food, constipation or diarrhoea. At least 6 out of 10 sufferers experience this form of migraine
- *migraine with aura* or classic migraine, includes visual disturbances as well as any or all of the symptoms of common migraine. Vision can be distorted with shimmering or flashing lights, strange zigzag shapes or blind spots.

Migraine without aura is often misdiagnosed as a tension headache. If you think your recurrent headache may be migraine, it is important to tell your doctor.

The exact cause of migraine is not fully understood. Attacks seem to be linked to chemical changes in the blood vessel walls and nerve cells within the skull. The most important chemical involved is called serotonin (5-hydroxytryptamine, or 5HT for short). Migraine headache occurs when blood vessels widen so that tissues become congested. Serotonin is in short supply during this phase. Some sufferers find their migraine is triggered by factors such as:

- stress or relief of stress (e.g. at the end of a long, trying week)
- physical fatigue or lack of sleep (e.g. due to hot sweats, insomnia)
- certain foods (e.g. cheese, alcohol – especially red wine, chocolate)
- extreme emotions (e.g. menopausal mood swings)
- hormonal changes (e.g. menstruation, oral contraceptive pill, menopausal symptoms).

Several different migraine treatments are now available, some over the counter, others by prescription only. While some people find simple analgesics control their symptoms, others need stronger medication. It's worth noting that digestion often shuts down during a migraine attack, so tablets are not always well absorbed. You may find that soluble or effervescent formulations suit you best.

There are two approaches to migraine treatment: the short-term relief of an acute attack, and long-term preventative treatment for people with frequent, disabling symptoms.

Short-term treatments contain simple painkillers such as

aspirin, paracetamol or codeine. Some also contain an anti-emetic to stop you feeling sick. The most modern treatments involve drugs that act on blood vessels in the brain in a similar way to serotonin (5HT – see above) to switch a migraine off in its early stages.

Long-term anti-migraine treatments come in several forms and if migraine has come on during the menopause, HRT may be suggested to help control your attacks. Several natural options are available, too (see Feverfew, Butterbur, Bowen Technique, Acupuncture).

Other Early Symptoms

A number of physical changes also occur in your body around the time of the menopause. These partly occur as a normal result of getting older, although they may be made worse by lack of oestrogen.

Wrinkles

Your skin tissues are sensitive to oestrogen and, after the menopause, your skin will become thinner, drier and more fragile. You will develop skin mottling and discoloration at a faster rate, and may develop broken capillaries (telangiectasia) as fine wine-red spidery tracings, especially on your face.

Every time your skin is exposed to the sun, it is damaged by ultraviolet rays. Over the years, this photodamage adds up to cause premature wrinkles and skin blemishes – a process known as photo-ageing or heliodermatitis. This is a normal part of the ageing process, although you can avoid some of the effects by minimizing the exposure of your skin to the sun. Solar ultraviolet radiation consists of UVA and

UVB rays. UVB causes sunburn and long-term changes responsible for skin ageing and skin cancer. UVA does not burn, but is responsible for photosensitivity reactions and also contributes to long-term photo-ageing.

As a result of photo-ageing, your skin cells are unable to regenerate normally and collagen fibres that provide under-lying skin support become matted, branched and twisted. Skin that is exposed to the sun over a long period of time eventually becomes inelastic, thickened, yellow, scaly, blem-ished and wrinkled.

Women who smoke cigarettes are five times more likely to suffer premature wrinkles than non-smokers, with the number of facial wrinkles directly linked to the number of cigarettes smoked.

There are three main types of skin wrinkle:

Crinkles Fine lines that disappear when skin is stretched. These are due to the breakdown of elastic fibres in your skin and start before the menopause, around the age of 30.

Glyphic wrinkles Accentuation of normal skin markings. Skin becomes yellowed and thickened where exposed to light – especially around the neck and eyes. These wrinkles become more pronounced after the menopause.

Linear furrows Grooves related to long-standing patterns of facial expression whose positions are determined in child-hood.

As well as wrinkles, ageing skin starts to develop other changes, including:

- **Age spots** – areas of pigmentation on skin that has been exposed to light over many years. These are often seen on the backs of the hands, face and neck

– *mottling*, irregular pigmentation in which, paradoxically, the number of skin pigment cells (melanocytes) is decreased
– *stellate pseudoscars*, small spots that are white, star shaped, and tend to appear after the age of 60
– *guttate hypomelanoses*, small round or angular spots that are pure white in colour and range in size from pinpoint to 15 mm across
– *ephelides*, small, brown marks which darken in the sun
– *senile lentigines*, darkened patches of skin that can be over 1 cm across. They are often dark brown, but can also be yellow, light brown or even black. A good intake of selenium helps to reduce development of age spots.

* **Pre-malignant lesions** that can progress to skin cancer if not treated. There are three types of skin cancer: malignant melanoma, basal cell carcinoma and squamous cell carcinoma. Malignant melanoma is now the second commonest cancer in women after cervical cancer. If you notice any skin lesions that are enlarging, itching, scabbing, bleeding, changing in colour or in any other way, always seek medical advice. Caught early, most skin cancers are readily curable.

Acne

Although acne is usually thought of as a teenage problem, it can affect anyone of any age and studies suggest that 5 per cent of people in their forties suffer from acne-like spots. In some cases, skin outbreaks can come on after the menopause due to hormonal imbalances that can occur when levels of testosterone increase as oestrogen levels fall.
Acne is thought to be triggered in some people by over

sensitivity of skin oil (sebaceous) glands to normal blood levels of the male hormone, testosterone. Although this hypersensitivity usually starts in the teens and switches off again within a few years, some people have trouble-free skin until their late twenties, early thirties or at the menopause, and then suddenly develop spots.

When oil glands are overactive, or under the influence of testosterone hormone, they produce a thick, oily secretion known as sebum. If you have a type of bacteria called *Propionibacterium acnes* living on your skin, it can produce enzymes that break the sebum down into a variety of fatty acids. These, plus other effects of the bacteria on immune chemicals in your skin, trigger inflammation and lead to classic acne lesions in those who are sensitive to them.

If your skin starts to flare up after the menopause, don't be afraid to consult your GP for treatment. Unfortunately, acne treatment needs patience as often, no benefits are seen for six to eight weeks after starting therapy. It is important to keep up with the treatment, however, as after two months of continued and regular use, improvements of around 20 per cent per month are common.

Hair Changes

Your hair is a good indicator of your general health and nutrition. It is often the first part of your body to show signs of ill health, or a dietary lack of vitamins, minerals or essential fatty acids. This is because, although hair is often thought of as a dead structure, its root – the hair follicle – is very much alive. The rate at which new hair cells are produced is second only to the speed at which new blood cells are made in the bone marrow. Your hair follicles therefore need a constant supply of nutrients for optimum health. Unlike the marrow, however, hair is a non-essential structure and your body preferentially diverts precious nutrient stores away from it in times of lack or stress. Research shows that levels of specific minerals laid down in the hair vary significantly with time – even from hour to hour.

The normal ageing process together with lack of oestrogen may make your hair feel drier and coarser than normal. You may also find that your hair is turning grey at a faster rate. Some women find that their skin and hair condition improve if they pay attention to their diet, take a good multinutrient supplement and increase their intake of essential fatty acids (found in evening primrose oil and fish oils).

FIVE TIPS FOR OPTIMUM HAIR HEALTH

1. Eat a healthy, balanced diet containing as many unrefined, wholefoods as possible. Wholegrains, fruit, vegetables and seeds are a rich source of vitamins, minerals and essential fatty acids that provide nourishment for hair roots and contribute to a healthy head of hair. Try not to eat erratically or to skip meals (especially breakfast) or the supply of nutrients to non-essential tissues such as hair follicles will be reduced. Try to eat something – for example a healthy snack such as fresh or dried fruit – at least every four hours. Hair has a high content of the tough, fibrous protein, keratin, which is made from amino acid building blocks obtained from your diet. Aim to eat a source of protein with every meal, such as poultry, fish, eggs, nuts or beans.

2. Reduce your salt intake – excess salt reduces hair follicle function and research shows that reducing salt intake can reduce hair loss and thinning by as much as 60 per cent.

3. Consider taking a good supplement designed for those aged 50 plus. Alternatively, choose one especially formulated for hair, skin and nails. You could also consider taking an evening primrose oil supplement (1000 mg per day). You will start to notice an improvement in the quality of your hair and nails within three months as new cells grow down, although as new hair only grows down at a rate of half an inch per month, it may take as long as a year for the overall improvement to show.

4. After the age of 25, the diameter of individual hairs naturally starts to decrease, especially in women. Although this often goes unnoticed, it can change the texture and body of your hair. By the age of 40, most people have finer hair with less body. At the same time, more follicles stay in their resting phase so less hair grows and the rate of growth decreases, resulting in progressive thinning. You can minimize this effect by massaging your scalp regularly with your fingers, at least once a week, and preferably every day. Try holding a handful of hair near the roots and vigorously moving the scalp back and forth and side to side to help loosen underlying tightness. Massage and scalp movement opens up the circulation and stimulates the flow of blood, oxygen and nutrients to the hair follicles.

5. The most important aspect of healthy hair is regular cleansing with shampoo. Contrary to popular belief, this does not dry out your hair but, if done properly, will remoisturize it. You may want to shampoo every day, selecting a product that suits your hair texture. Fine, limp hair needs body-building products; wavy, medium hair can use products labelled 'normal' while curly or frizzy hair needs moisturizing products. Chemically treated hair needs

extra moisture and deep conditioning. Always use a conditioner after shampooing, as this will de-tangle and smooth hair shafts. Thoroughly rinse your hair – for longer than you think necessary – to remove excess shampoo and conditioner which can cause hair to look dull.

INCREASE IN FACIAL HAIR

Excess, unwanted female facial hair is common, especially from middle age onward. A quarter of all women have noticeable hair on their face. As levels of oestrogen fall around the time of the menopause, the effects of testosterone hormone become more pronounced without the feminizing effects of oestrogen to counter-balance them. As a result, facial hair increases. By the age of 65, 40 per cent of women have a noticeable moustache and 10 per cent sprout hair on their chins. This is not due to any medically significant hormonal imbalance, but to the changing balance between masculine and feminine hormones.

The best way to cope with unwanted hair is by using depilatory creams, plucking, epilation or waxing. For a more permanent method, you could have a course of electrolysis, laser or sound wave therapy. These treatments only work on growing hair, however, not on follicles in their rest phase, so you may need another course a few months later as resting follicles start to activate.

Contrary to popular belief, shaving does not thicken hair or make it grow faster. It does however slice off the tapered tip of the hair shaft to leave a flattened stubble that quickly becomes noticeable again.

Tiredness

Tiredness and lack of energy affect as many as one in three

women during the menopausal years. It tends up creep up on you, making you feel washed out and exhausted for much of the time. These symptoms seem to be linked with oestrogen withdrawal as they usually improve with hormone replacement therapy, especially in women suffering more severe hot flushes. Minor vitamin and mineral deficiencies may be involved, and women taking a good multinutrient supplement – including sensible levels of B group vitamins – usually notice an improvement. (See also Kelp, Iodine, Ginseng, Guarana, Co-enzyme Q10.)

Aches and Pains

Aches and pains are common during the time of oestrogen withdrawal. Headaches become more frequent and your joints and muscles may stiffen and hurt. It is possible that these symptoms are related to changes in blood flow and circulation in musculoskeletal tissues. Symptoms often improve with hormone replacement therapy. See Omega-3 fish oils, Evening Primrose Oil, Glucosamine, Chondroitin and MSM-Sulphur.

Early Emotional Symptoms of the Menopause

Many women find the emotional symptoms of the menopause more troublesome than the physical symptoms. Emotional symptoms can occur at any time around the menopause, but tend to come on before your periods have finally ended. If left untreated, these symptoms tend to be worse during the first one or two years and then improve as your body adjusts to lower levels of oestrogen. The average duration for emotional menopausal symptoms seems to be around three and a half years. One in ten women get over them within six months, while one in five women are not really troubled by them at all. Emotional symptoms that can accompany the menopause include:

- difficulty sleeping
- strange dreams
- changes in sensations, including vision, smell and taste
- fuzzy feelings in the head
- early morning waking
- low mood
- crying for no obvious reason
- sudden, unexplained anger
- mood swings
- increased anxiety and depression
- panic attacks
- loss of self-esteem
- inability to cope
- irritability
- poor memory
- difficulty concentrating
- low sex drive.

Most women only experience a few of these symptoms. Many women describe their menopausal mood swings as similar to those occurring before their periods as part of pre-menstrual syndrome. Not surprisingly, low mood seems to be more common in women who also suffer from more severe physical symptoms. I have described in more detail below the worst of the emotional symptoms.

Irritability

Irritability seems to be linked with falling oestrogen levels which affect higher centres of the brain. This may be more common in women who experience irritability with premenstrual syndrome, although some women who have never had problems before develop cyclical mood swings at the menopause similar to those occurring in PMS. In some cases, irritability is linked with lack of sleep, especially rapid eye movement (REM) sleep. Irritability usually gets better on its own, although HRT or complementary therapies can help enormously. Irritability can also be due to low blood sugar levels. It is worth drinking a glass of freshly squeezed orange juice for an instant lift, followed by a crispbread, slice of wholemeal bread, rice cake or banana to see if this helps (see food cravings below).

Mood swings

Some women going through the menopause experience alarming mood swings, going from happy to sad, or suffering from anxiety and panic attacks for no obvious reason. In contrast, other women find that once their periods stop, they no longer suffer from premenstrual syndrome and actually feel more emotionally stable than before. While it is easy to blame emotional changes on falling hormone levels, this time of life is also one where you may be experiencing other stresses, such as caring for elderly relatives, offspring leaving home, a husband in a mid-life crisis and your own changing self-image.

If your mood swings are pronounced, you may find it helps to take a regular energetic form of exercise such as going for a brisk walk or even taking up gentle jogging to get fit. Exercise releases chemicals in the brain that help to lift your mood and keep you on a more even keel. The exercise needs to be brisk enough to leave you slightly breathless and to raise your pulse to between 100–120 beats per minute.

Anxiety

Anxiety affects 5 per cent of the population and is associated with feelings of apprehension, dread and impending doom. It can cause physical symptoms similar to those caused by stress, such as:

- restlessness
- palpitations
- tremor
- flushing
- dizziness
- over breathing (hyperventilation)
- loose bowels
- sweating (which makes hot flushes worse)
- muscle tension
- difficulty sleeping.

In most cases, anxiety linked with other menopausal symptoms is self-limiting and gets better over the course of a few weeks without any specific treatment. Symptoms are usually made worse by drinking caffeine or alcohol, however, and it is worth avoiding these.

It is now thought that anxiety and panic attacks are linked with over breathing. As a result, you inhale too much oxygen and exhale too much carbon dioxide causing an imbalance of respiratory gases, which in turn makes your blood too alkaline. As well as triggering symptoms of dizziness, faintness and 'pins and needles' in the face and limbs, over breathing sends messages to the brain that you are under stress and keeps the body on Red Alert. Habitual hyperventilators may also experience chest pains, palpitations, sleep disturbances and other physical symptoms as well as anxiety. If you feel anxiety coming on, consciously try to slow and control your breathing – if necessary, try the old trick of breathing in and out of a brown paper bag as this helps you to breathe back in some of the carbon dioxide you have exhaled.

See Meditation, Valerian for how they can help alleviate these symptoms.

Tearfulness and Depression

Few people are blessed with a happy mood all the time. One day you may feel cheerful, energetic and lively, while the next you feel gloomy, listless and withdrawn for no obvious reason. These mood swings are a normal part of everyday life. But sometimes they can get out of hand – and if your mood swings too low, mild depression can occur.

Tearfulness is common around the time of the menopause, and is linked with falling oestrogen levels. While mild cases usually improve rapidly with close support from family and friends, taking regular exercise, and using beneficial alternative treatments (see St John's Wort), in some cases your mood can fall even lower until you are suffering from a full-blown depressive illness.

Depression occurs when the level of various chemical messengers in the brain become unbalanced. These chemicals – known as neurotransmitters – are responsible for passing messages from one brain cell to another by passing across the tiny gap (synapse) between each brain cell. Once across the gap, they trigger an electrical response in the next brain cell to increase its activity. After it has done its job, the neurotransmitter is then reabsorbed into the cell that released it and broken down for re-cycling. If your neuro-transmitter levels fall too low, messages are not passed from one brain cell to another properly and mild depression occurs; your brain cells are not being kick-started like they should be.

Overall, women are twice as likely to suffer depression than men – your life-time risk of developing a severe depres-sive illness is between 20–26 per cent while for men it is 8–12 per cent. While it is traditionally believed that female depression is most likely to occur between the ages of 35–55 years – i.e. in women approaching and just past the menopause – recent research suggests that female depression is no more common in your forties or fifties than earlier or later in life. For women who do develop depression around the time of the menopause, however, hormonal changes are the most usual trigger – to the extent that a psychiatrist seeing a depressed woman at this time of life is likely to suggest treatment with hormone replacement therapy rather than an anti-depressant medication. Some researchers now believe that low mood is due to sleep disturbances – espe-cially lack of REM sleep – linked with falling oestrogen levels or brought on by other menopausal problems such as night sweats and insomnia.

Symptoms of mild depression can include:

- anxiety
- agitation
- tiredness during the day
- headache

- loss of self-esteem/confidence
- comfort eating
- feeling sad
- crying for no apparent reason.

Symptoms of a more serious depression include:

- lethargy and listlessness with loss of interest in life
- loss of concentration
- continual weepiness for no obvious reason
- feeling slowed up both physically and mentally
- loss of sex drive
- difficulty in sleeping
- early morning waking between 2.00 and 5.00 a.m.
- loss of appetite with weight loss
- feeling of worthlessness
- feeling that life isn't worth living.

Serious Depression

If you have any of the symptoms of more serious depression, it is important to seek medical help before you get any worse. One in two cases of depression needing medical treatment remain undiagnosed causing countless sadness and despair.

The symptoms are due to an imbalance of chemical transmitters in the brain, which can be made worse by falling hormone levels. While in most cases the symptoms will eventually get better on their own, this can take months or even years. Drug treatment with antidepressants – which are not addictive – can boost levels of brain chemicals and help you start feeling better within a matter of days. In most cases, antidepressant tablets will need to be taken for at least three to six months before slowly stopping them. Alternatively, treatment with HRT may be suggested if this is thought to be your main problem.

Difficulty Concentrating and Poor Memory

Your memory is a personal storehouse of information. Around the time of the menopause, it is natural for your memory to become less like a filing cabinet and more like a sieve. You have three main types of memory:

- *sensory memory,* which stores information for only a split second
- *short-term memory,* which stores facts for up to 5 minutes
- *long-term memory,* which can store facts for a lifetime.

Researchers are still unsure exactly how memory is stored, although one part of the brain in particular – the hippocampus – seems to be important in processing and storing long-term information. It is thought that new connections (synapses) are laid down between brain cells (neurones), and that new protein molecules are made to store information. It is possible that spare genetic material – DNA not being used to hold the genetic code – is involved, or that electrical circuits play a part.

Falling hormone levels affect your ability to store information for any length of time. It is worth developing a few tricks to improve your memory, such as writing notes to yourself on sticky pads and leaving them in obvious places. Supplements such as Ginkgo biloba or lecithin can help, as can using aromatherapy oils (e.g. Basil) to boost your clarity of thought.

Food Cravings

Appetite, or the desire for food, is a very personal phenomenon. It is influenced by sensations of hunger but can
produce insidious, niggling desires to eat even when your
stomach is groaning with food. Appetite is regulated by two
areas in the brain – the *feeding centre* and the *satiety centre*.
There is also a *thirst* centre regulating your intake of fluids.
On top of this, the presence of food in certain parts of the
gut also releases hormones that switch off your desire to eat.

Despite these regulations, some people can still eat through
feelings of satiety, because of especially strong appetite signals
– or food cravings. These tend to become more common at
times of hormone fluctuation, e.g. just before a period, and
around the time of the menopause – probably due to the
effects of hormone receptors in these parts of the brain. When
you eat carbohydrates, two things occur:

- insulin is secreted by the pancreas
- tiny amounts of a chemical called serotonin are released
  in the brain.

Both insulin and serotonin play a major role in controlling
your eating behaviour and food choices. Insulin is a hormone
that allows blood glucose to enter cells and provide a source
of energy. Usually, just enough insulin is secreted after eating
to cope with the exact amount of carbohydrate ingested. If
you produce too much insulin, however, blood sugar levels
may fall too quickly and you will experience food cravings,
irritability and even feelings of faintness.

It is only when your insulin levels start to fall that release
of serotonin is triggered in the brain. Serotonin is a neuro-
transmitter. It relays messages across important nerve

connections (synapses) and has a number of different functions. These include influencing appetite, the way you select certain foods and triggers feelings of having eaten enough. Serotonin also gives you a chemical high that makes you feel good and can help to lift depression. Low levels of serotonin have been linked experimentally to over-eating and food cravings and can occur around the time of the menopause.

Follow a wholefood diet with plenty of fresh fruit and vegetables and complex carbohydrates and avoid table sugar as much as possible.

When a snack attack occurs:

- Eat some carbohydrate, e.g. a slice of wholemeal bread, a couple of plain crispbread or rice cakes – but avoid carbohydrate linked with extra fat such as a sausage roll, a cream cake or doughnut
- When you eat, chew slowly and pause between each mouthful, so that the metabolic and emotional effects triggered by eating – and which tell you that you are full – have time to click in before you have eaten too much.
- If the craving continues, drink a glass of sparkling mineral water fortified with the juice of half a lemon or try cleaning your teeth slowly with a strongly flavoured, tingling toothpaste
- Go for a brisk walk or take another energetic form of exercise
- Eat a piece of fruit – a banana is particularly good
- Take a vitamin and mineral supplement containing iron and zinc.

The next chapter takes us on to the next phase of symptoms related to the menopause.

5
Medium-term Effects

After a while, low oestrogen levels cause some body tissues to thin down and become less elastic, producing medium-term effects of the menopause. These tend to come on within five years after you have experienced your last period, and can last indefinitely without treatment, and may worsen with time. They are not always troublesome, however.

As we saw at the end of Chapter 3, there are a variety of possible medium-term symptoms of the menopause, the most important of which are described here.

Thinning of Vaginal Tissues

Thinning of vaginal tissues is known as atrophic vaginitis (AV) or urogenital ageing. Symptoms of AV, which can cause itching, burning and urinary discomfort, are often misdiagnosed as infection, and by the time most women are referred to see a gynaecologist, they have often already received inappropriate anti-fungal and antibiotic treatments, when what you need is a localized form of oestrogen replacement therapy. Even where infection is present in a post-menopausal woman, the root of the problem is lack of oestrogen. Oestrogen replacement restores the natural pH balance of the vagina, encourages the healthy, beneficial, probiotic bacteria (lactobacilli) to recolonize the vagina, which reduces susceptibility to infections such as Candida. Many women have oestrogen deficient vaginitis complicated by a chemical vaginitis from the self use of lotions and creams such as TCP and Germolene.

The main criteria for diagnosing AV include vaginal dryness, painful intercourse and vaginal irritation, with symptoms of soreness and itch for which no infection can be found.

Many women only respond to local oestrogen treatment, rather than taking oral HRT. Local treatments available include oestrogen cream (with an applicator), vaginal tablets, pessaries and a vaginal ring. Local treatment has the advantage that very little is absorbed, so that side-effects are uncommon (although there is a ring available – Menoring 50 – that delivers a full HRT dose and which can be used to treat hot flushes and other such symptoms in a woman who has had a hysterectomy).

The vaginal oestrogen ring (Estring) is popular, as it is convenient and non-messy to use – many find long-term treatment with creams and pessaries messy and unacceptable. Once in place, the ring delivers a small, steady dose of oestrogen exactly where it is needed. There is no vaginal discharge, apart from the natural lubrication encouraged by oestrogen replacement.

The ring is left in place for three months, and then replaced – either by a doctor, nurse or by yourself if you are happy to do this. Some women prefer to remove the ring before making love and then re-insert it afterwards themselves, although this is not usually necessary, as nine out of ten partners are unable to detect it during sex. If the ring falls out initially because you are too dry, an oestrogen cream can be used for two weeks, then Estring can be refitted. This makes insertion and retention much easier.

If vaginal dryness continues, you should see your doctor. There is a condition called Sjögren's Syndrome in which the eyes, mouth, nose, throat or vagina can become overly dry due to the immune system attacking the normal lubricating glands. Nine out of ten sufferers are women, mostly over the age of 30. If you have also noticed dry, gritty eyes, this condition is a possibility, and you should consult your doctor for investigation. It is not particularly serious, but you will need treatment with lubricants such as artificial tears and saliva.

Reduced Sensation in the Skin, Nipples and Genitals

The skin responds to oestrogen levels, and many women find that skin all over their body – including the nipples and genitals – becomes less sensitive as oestrogen levels fall. One study found that six out of ten postmenopausal women noticed skin numbness so that caresses from their partner were no longer enjoyable. Not surprisingly, nine out of ten of these women found this sensory loss interfered with their enjoyment of sex. See Chapter 14.

Changing Body Shape

Many women are distressed to realize their body shape is changing as they grow older. As well as a spreading waistline, you may notice that your breasts shrink, your hips lose their rounded curves, and you gain weight in unusual places such as the upper back and behind the knees. These changes are partly due to lack of oestrogen and partly to lack of exercise. They can often be minimized by following a healthy diet, maintaining a healthy weight and taking regular exercise to help tone muscles all over the body so they retain their bulk (See Chapter 11).

Urinary Symptoms

Urinary discomfort due to stress incontinence – the leakage of urine during physical exertion such as coughing, sneezing, walking or even just walking – is thought to affect at least 60 per cent of women after the menopause. Some cases are mild with only slight damping, but a few women experience a significant loss of bladder control. Unfortunately, half of all sufferers never consult their doctor either through embarrassment or a mistaken belief that nothing can be done. In fact, seven out of ten cases of stress incontinence are curable with the right treatment.

Stress incontinence is due to weakness of the pelvic floor muscles, so that the neck of the bladder is no longer properly supported allowing it to sag. This causes the opening around the urethra (tube through which urine flows from the bladder to the outside world) to open. Sometimes, the bladder also bulges into the front of the vagina, causing a pouching known as a cystocoele. Most cases are linked with previous childbirth, especially if you have had large babies or many children.

Lack of pelvic floor support places strain on sphincters keeping the bladder and urethral openings closed. A sudden increase in intra-abdominal pressure, as happens during lifting, coughing, laughing, sneezing or running, then results in urine leaking out. Many sufferers cut down on their fluid intake in an attempt to dry things up, but this only makes matters worse. Your urine becomes concentrated, more irritant and is also more likely to produce a detectable smell. Even if you have problems with leaking urine, it is important to maintain an adequate fluid intake of at least two to three litres a day.

When you consult your doctor, a water sample will be analysed to rule out any infection (cystitis) and you will be gently examined to assess your pelvic organs and look for any prolapse. In some cases, further investigation is needed to measure your urinary flow, bladder pressure and to see whether your bladder muscles are over-sensitive – a condition known as irritable bladder. If you have pure stress incontinence, however, you will usually be referred to a physiotherapist or incontinence advisor to learn pelvic floor exercises – these produce a dramatic improvement in 30–70 per cent of women.

If you are able and willing to take hormone replacement therapy, this will help return your vaginal tissues to their plumper, more moist, pre-menopausal state and will help to cure mild cases of incontinence, as well as increasing the chance of success with exercises or surgery. If you don't want to take full HRT tablets or patches, you may benefit from localized treatment in the form of an oestrogen vaginal ring or oestrogen vaginal tablets which supply oestrogen locally to tissues with little being absorbed into the circulation. The older oestrogen creams are less acceptable as they are messy, some hormone is absorbed into the circulation – which is not always desirable – and many women soon stop using them.

Pelvic Floor Exercises

Pelvic floor exercises aim to strengthen and build up the muscles supporting your bladder and urethra so that leakage of urine no longer occurs. There are two types of muscle fibre involved:

- *slow twitch fibres*, which need multiple repeated contractions to retrain them
- *fast twitch fibres*, which need maximum 'squeeze' effort to retrain them.

Once you have learned how to do the exercises, you need to practice them several times a day, little and often – some contractions will be quick short ones, while others will last up to 10 seconds. These exercises can be done almost anywhere, as they are virtually undetectable.

A simple exercise is to pull up your front and back passages tightly as if trying to stop your bowels and bladder from opening. Hold tight for a count of four and repeat this every hour, increasing in frequency as you find them easier to do.

Some women find it difficult to identify the muscles involved, in which case you may be shown how to insert one or two fingers into your vagina so that you can practice squeezing these until you can recognise which are the relevant muscles. Training devices, such as the Pelvic Toner, are also available, which you insert and squeeze to tone up the pelvic floor.

You will be advised to repeat these exercises regularly throughout the day (e.g. ten sets of ten) and should start to notice an improvement within three months. Continued progress should follow over several months. It is important to persevere – exercising at regular intervals every day – as progress can be slow but sure. Once you have started doing the exercises regularly, you can test the strength of your pelvic floor muscles once a month by jumping, running or skipping on the spot to see if you leak any urine. If you seem to reach a point where no further improvement occurs, however, consult your doctor for further advice.

Tips to improve stress incontinence

- Pull in your pelvic floor muscles before coughing, sneezing or lifting
- Avoid standing for long periods of time
- Lose any excess weight, which puts unwanted extra pressure on pelvic floor muscles
- Eat plenty of fibre and drink plenty of fluids to avoid constipation – straining to open your bowels will weaken your pelvic muscles
- Avoid carrying heavy weights
- Make sure your bladder is completely empty after each visit to the bathroom
- Take regular exercise to tone up muscles throughout your body.

Other Treatments

If pelvic floor exercises alone do not solve the problem, a number of other measures can help:

- physiotherapists can strengthen your pelvic floor muscles using a tiny electric current – two electric pads are placed on the perineum (tissue between the vagina and anus) to stimulate the muscles at regular intervals

- you can wear weighted cones inside the vagina for ten to 15 minutes twice a day – weights vary from 5 g to 60 g and this will help to tighten and tone your muscles, which have to contract to hold the cone in place
- a urethral balloon device can be fitted into the neck of the bladder with a reusable applicator – the balloon in the tip is then inflated to block urine leakage.

Collagen Injections Some surgeons treat stress incontinence by injecting collagen around the urethra and neck of the bladder under local anaesthetic – usually two injections are given, one on either side of the urethra. The collagen increases tissue bulk at the neck of the bladder and helps to keep the bladder opening closed. Before the collagen is injected around your bladder, you will need to have a small injection of collagen into your skin to make sure you are not allergic to the preparation. Studies show that over 80 per cent of women notice a marked improvement, with 60 per cent becoming totally dry. Less than 4 per cent of women notice little or no benefit. Two years on, almost 70 per cent of women treated were still improved and 50 per cent dry. Most women need to have the bladder collagen implants repeated at occasional intervals, as the collagen is slowly absorbed into the body.

Surgery for Stress Incontinence Traditional surgery for improving stress incontinence has a 95 per cent success rate. It involves stitching a nylon sling under the neck of the bladder to provide support, tightening loose tissues and sometimes taking in vaginal tucks (colporrhaphy) if the bladder or rectum are prolapsing through the vaginal walls. This tightens the vagina, as well as helping to support the bladder. As a bonus, many women find this also improves their sex life.

A new technique, known as the Tension-Free Vaginal Tape operation, can now be performed in just 30 minutes as a day case surgery under local anaesthetic or spinal anaesthesia. This allows the surgeon to adjust the tape position to achieve the right level of urinary control for each individual patient. You can usually leave hospital the same day as the level of post-operative pain is low, and follow up studies show that 90 per cent of women are cured or have significant improved symptoms even five years after surgery.

Sometimes, prolapse of the uterus makes it difficult to correct stress incontinence unless the womb is removed. If your family is complete, a vaginal hysterectomy may be the best option. This can be performed at the same time as supporting the neck of the bladder and – as the womb is removed through the vagina – has the advantage of not leaving an abdominal scar.

Increased Tendency to Bruising

Easy bruising is common in older people due to increased fragility of skin and blood vessels (known as Easy Bruising Syndrome). If excessive, it is important to see your doctor, as you may need a blood test to investigate the possible of a bleeding tendency. Occasionally, lack of vitamin K can be a cause of easy bruising in older people, and you should ask your doctor's advice about taking supplements containing these. General skin quality can be improved by taking evening primrose oil capsules (at least 1 g daily), plus bilberry or red vine leaf extracts, which help to strengthen small blood vessels. While many older people suffer from an increased tendency to bruising, the menopause can exacerbate the problem because of the thinning of blood vessels of the tissues that support them.

6
Long-term Effects

A number of serious diseases and conditions – including osteo-porosis, female coronary heart disease (CHD), circulatory problems and Alzheimer's – are associated with the meno-pause. These debilitating and often life-threatening conditions bring misery to many women.

Long-term problems due to lack of oestrogen tend not to appear for at least five years after your last period. Oestrogen has lots of important effects on many different parts of your body, including your arteries, bones and brain. As your oestrogen levels fall, your metabolism starts to change, which can lead to:

- raised levels of a type of blood fat called LDL cholesterol
- hardening and furring up of the arteries
- raised levels of a potentially harmful amino acid called homocysteine
- an increased risk of Cardiac and Metabolic Syndrome X
- an increased risk of dementia, including Alzheimer's disease

- an increased risk of high blood pressure, coronary heart disease and stroke
- an increased risk of osteoporosis.

The risk of many of these problems can be reduced by adopting a healthy diet and lifestyle. Taking HRT – either natural or prescribed forms – may also help. Blood fat levels and hardening and furring up of the arteries are discussed in this chapter, along with Syndrome X and memory problems. Osteoporosis is discussed separately in Chapter 7.

Raised Cholesterol Levels

Once dietary fats are absorbed from your intestines into the circulation, they are transported in the blood as lipoproteins, in which they are bound to special carrier proteins. Once they reach your liver, the fats are processed, packaged to different types of carrier proteins and passed out into the circulation again for further distribution around your body. There are two main types of circulating cholesterol:

- low-density liporotein (LDL) cholesterol, which is linked with hardening and furring up of artery walls, high blood pressure and coronary heart disease
- high-density lipoprotein (HDL) cholesterol, that protects against atherosclerosis and CHD by transporting LDL-cholesterol away from the arteries for metabolism.

It is not so much your total blood cholesterol level that is important when it comes to atherosclerosis, but the ratio between beneficial HDL cholesterol and harmful LDL cholesterol. Research shows that for every 1 per cent rise in beneficial HDL cholesterol, there is a corresponding fall in the risk of CHD of as much as 2 per cent. This seems to be due to reversed cholesterol transport in which HDL moves LDL cholesterol away from the tissues and back towards the liver.

If you are told you have a raised blood cholesterol level, it is therefore important to know whether it is your LDL or HDL cholesterol that is high. If most of the lipids are in the form of LDL cholesterol, with low HDL levels, your risk of CHD is significantly increased. Ideally, the total cholesterol level should be less than 5 mmol/l, with LDL cholesterol less than 3 mmol/l.

Raised levels of LDL cholesterol become more common in women after the menopause. This is because oestrogen has beneficial effects on the circulation, helping to maintain healthy blood fat levels and to maintain elastic arteries.

Raised Homocysteine Levels

Homocysteine is an amino acid formed in the body from the breakdown of the dietary amino acid, methionine. Homocysteine is highly reactive and high levels can damage artery walls to the extent that a raised blood homocysteine level snow recognized as an important risk factor for developing coronary heart disease and stroke. It has been estimated that 10 per cent of the risk of coronary artery disease in the general population is, in fact, due to homocysteine.

As it is so toxic, homocysteine levels are normally tightly controlled by three different enzymes that convert homocysteine to cysteine – a safe end product used by cells for growth. Two of the three enzymes that control homocysteine levels depend on folic acid, vitamin B6 and vitamin B12 for their activity. Women who do not obtain enough folic acid or B vitamins for optimal enzyme function will have a raised homocysteine level and an increased risk of circulatory problems that may be three times higher than normal, especially after the menopause. Unfortunately, lack of folic acid seems to be common and may affect as many as 50 per cent of people.

One in ten people also inherit genetic mutations that can decrease the activity of any one of the three controlling enzymes to raise homocysteine levels, while one in 160,000 people have extremely high levels, with 30 times the risk of premature heart disease. After the menopause, some women are also less able to process homocysteine, so levels build up to increase the risk of osteoporosis and coronary heart disease.

The risks associated with a raised homocysteine level are comparable to those of an abnormally raised cholesterol level, but are more easily corrected through dietary means. Taking a vitamin and mineral supplement providing as little as 200 g of folic acid per day (the EU RDA) is effective in lowering moderately raised plasma homocysteine levels. High levels of homocysteine can be reduced by taking folic acid supplements supplying 400 mcg to 650 mcg per day. Women with a family or personal history of coronary heart disease may wish to consider taking supplements of at least 400 mcg folic acid daily, especially after the menopause, to help reduce some of the long-term effects of oestrogen deprivation.

In the UK, some food packagings have special flashes to show they contain folic acid – these were designed for pregnant women whose need for folic acid is significantly increased, but are also helpful for people with increased risk of heart disease. Folic acid should usually be taken together with vitamin B12. This is because lack of vitamin B12 (which leads to damage of the nervous system, especially the spinal cord) is masked by taking folic acid supplements (as this prevents the occurrence of pernicious anaemia, which usually allows lack of vitamin B12 to be detected).

Hardening and Furring up of the Arteries

Hardening and furring up of the arteries – known as atherosclerosis – becomes more common after the menopause once oestrogen levels fall, as oestrogen receptors found in blood vessel walls help to keep them elastic. Oestrogen also affects the way dietary fats are metabolized to raise blood levels of beneficial fats and lower levels of harmful ones.

Oestrogen helps to:

- Lower total cholesterol levels
- Lower low-density lipoprotein (LDL) cholesterol
- Increase protective high-density lipoprotein (HDL) cholesterol
- Optimize processing of homocysteine
- Protect circulating fats from oxidation.

The roots of atherosclerosis start early in life, usually in your teens. Normal wear-and-tear to blood vessel walls damages artery linings. Some of this damage is triggered by oxidation of dietary polyunsaturated fats. This damage is hastened by factors such as smoking cigarettes, lack of dietary anti-oxidants (e.g. vitamins C, E), raised homocysteine levels and high blood pressure. When damage occurs, small cell fragments (platelets) in the bloodstream stick to the arterial lining to form a tiny clot. The platelets then release chemicals that stimulate growth of underlying smooth muscle cells in the artery wall. Under normal circumstances, this would lead to healing – but if your blood contains raised levels of oxidised fat molecules, the proliferating smooth muscle cells start to accumulate excessive amounts of fat.

At the same time, a type of immune cell known as macrophages ingests circulating fats that it recognizes as foreign. The most popular theory is that macrophages mistake oxidized dietary fats for invading bacteria. Once over-loaded with these ingested fats, the macrophages try to leave the circulation, but become trapped in artery walls where smooth muscle cells are proliferating. This sets up an inflammatory reaction that attracts more macrophages into the area, so the process accelerates. As a result, fatty swellings known as atheromatous (*porridge-like*) plaques build up which initially form fatty streaks along artery walls.

As time progresses, further damage to an atheromatous plaque results in ulceration of its surface. More platelets stick to the damaged area to form a larger clot (thrombus). The platelets trigger the same process over again and typically, a layered build-up of clot and fatty substances develops, slowly narrowing the coronary artery. At the same time, the under-lying middle layer of the artery starts to degenerate, loses its elasticity (especially after the menopause) and becomes hard-ened and fibrous. Over a period of time, this can cause a significant fall in blood supply to peripheral body tissues as well as the heart.

Atherosclerosis can affect arteries throughout the body – the only arteries that seem to escape are those supplying the lungs, which contain a relatively low blood pressure. If widespread, hardening and furring of the arteries leads to high blood pressure, damage to internal organs (e.g. kidneys) and poor peripheral circulation (e.g. reduced blood supply to the legs). If the process impairs blood supply in the brain, gradual death of brain cells may lead to senility, while sudden blockage of a brain artery – or rupture of a damaged vessel – will cause a stroke.

In some cases, an atherosclerotic plaque eventually fractures, leading to haemorrhage within the blood vessel wall. This triggers a rapid build-up of thrombocytes to form a clot large enough to suddenly block the artery and cut off the blood supply to part of the heart muscle. This causes a heart attack (coronary thrombosis). The clot may also break off and wander around the bloodstream (thrombo-embolus) to impact elsewhere, commonly in the lungs (pulmonary embolus) or the brain (stroke).

Although this sounds frightening, there are several diet and lifestyle measures you can take to help maintain a healthy circulation after the menopause. See Chapter 8, Diet and the Menopause and Chapter 11, Exercise and Lifestyle for detailed suggestions.

Blood Pressure

Everyone needs a certain blood pressure (BP) to keep blood moving around their body and maintain their circulation. Normal BP varies naturally throughout the day and night, going up and down in response to your emotions and level of activity. If you have high blood pressure, however, your BP will remain consistently high, even when you are asleep. The pressure in your arteries at any time depends on a number of factors, including the volume of fluid inside your circulation, how hard your heart is pumping, how constricted or dilated your blood vessels are and how elastic they are.

The highest pressure in the arteries occur when the heart beats to push blood through the circulation. This is known as the *systolic* pressure, as it is due to contraction (systole) of the heart. As the heart rests between beats (diastole) the blood pressure falls to its lowest point, known as the *diastolic* pressure. In general, if the heart pumps more strongly, it is systolic pressure that goes up, while in a reduction in elasticity of the arteries (e.g. due to the hardening and furring up of atherosclerosis) it is the diastolic pressure that is most affected.

BP is measured according to the length of a column of mercury it can support. Blood pressure is therefore expressed in millimetres of mercury (mmHg). BP is written down as the higher pressure (systole) over the lower figure (diastole).

Hypertension

As many as one in five adults have high blood pressure, known medically as hypertension. Hypertension is diagnosed when systolic pressure is consistently greater than 140 mmHg and diastolic pressure consistently greater than 90 mmHg.

Unfortunately, people with high blood pressure usually notice few symptoms. As a result, it creeps up on you without any obvious warning. Even if your blood pressure is dangerously high, you may feel relatively well. If symptoms do occur, they tend to be non-specific, such as headache or getting up at night to pass urine more often than normal. Your blood pressure has to be severely raised before you develop dizziness or visual disturbances. It is therefore a good idea for adults to have their blood pressure checked on a regular basis, every year or so – especially if high blood pressure runs in their family. If left untreated, high blood pressure will worsen atherosclerosis, and damage blood vessels throughout the body, causing numerous complications.

Women are relatively protected against high blood pressure until the menopause, due to the beneficial effects of natural oestrogen on the circulation. Often, eating a healthy diet, losing any excess weight and remaining physically active can prevent high blood pressure developing in later life. If it does develop, it usually responds well to changes in diet and lifestyle, although anti-hypertensive drugs may be needed, too.

Female Coronary Heart Disease (CHD)

Coronary heart disease is often thought of as a male problem, yet it accounts for the death of as many as one in four women, and kills more women each year than cancer of the cervix, uterus and ovaries combined.

One advantage that women do have over men is that the female hormone, oestrogen, helps to protect against CHD until after the menopause. Oestrogen acts on tissues in the artery walls to keep them elastic and also affects the way dietary fats are metabolized to raise blood levels of beneficial fats and lower levels of harmful ones. As a result, it helps to discourage hardening and furring up of the arteries (atherosclerosis). Once you reach the menopause however, and your oestrogen levels fall, you lose this protective effect and women rapidly develop the same risk of CHD as men.

How Heart Disease Develops

The heart is made up of a special type of muscle (myocardium) that beats continuously and consumes a large amount of oxygen. It receives blood from two main vessels, the left and right coronary arteries which join up in places to help safeguard against blockage of one or the other.

Coronary heart disease occurs when one or both of the coronary arteries become narrowed or blocked, usually through a process of hardening and furring up called atherosclerosis so that the heart muscle no longer receives all the blood it needs. Tissue that is not receiving enough oxygen triggers a type of heart pain known as angina, which is usually:

- felt as a pain or discomfort behind the chest bone
- tight and crushing – like a bear hug
- described as spreading through the chest and may radiate up into the neck, jaw or down the left arm
- brought on by exertion and relieved by rest.

If heart muscle cells die due to prolonged oxygen starvation, a heart attack occurs. Heart attack pain is similar to angina, but:

- lasts longer
- is more intense
- is usually accompanied by sweating, paleness and breathlessness
- can come on at any time and is unrelieved by rest.

Sudden chest pain should always be taken seriously and medical assistance sought without delay.

CHD Risk Factors

A risk factor is anything that increases your chance of a particular illness. Over 200 different risk factors have been linked with CHD, although not all of them are proven. For women, the risk factors that are most closely associated with atherosclerosis and having a heart attack include:

- increasing age after the menopause
- having a family history of coronary heart disease
- smoking cigarettes
- having uncontrolled high blood pressure
- eating a poor diet containing a high percentage of fat and not enough fresh fruit and vegetables
- being overweight or obese
- having abnormally raised blood fat levels (cholesterol, triglycerides)
- having abnormally raised homocysteine levels
- not taking enough exercise
- drinking excessive amounts of alcohol
- having poorly controlled diabetes
- having high stress levels.

Modifiable Risk Factors

Although there is very little you can do to slow the ageing process or change the genes you have inherited, you can modify your lifestyle to reduce your risk of coronary heart disease. It is never too late to make these changes, even if you have reached the menopause and feel unhealthy. Your risk factors can be modified by:

- stopping smoking
- losing any excess weight
- exercising for at least 20 minutes, three times a week or more
- eating a healthy diet

- cutting back on salt intake to help reduce your blood pressure
- drinking no more than two to three units of alcohol per day
- avoiding excessive stress
- having regular check-ups to assess your blood pressure, cholesterol levels and general cardiovascular fitness
- increasing your intake of soy and other foods rich in isoflavones (see pages 149–50).

It is surprising what a difference these steps can make. Computer analysis of many trials suggests that for each risk factor you modify, your risk of CHD is lowered as follows:

Factor modified	Reduction in risk of CHD
Stopping smoking	50–70 per cent lower risk within five years
Exercise	45 per cent lower risk for those who exercise regularly
Losing excess weight	35–55 per cent lower risk for those who maintain a healthy weight
Keeping alcohol intake within healthy limits	25–45 per cent lower risk for those drinking two to three units per day
Controlling high blood pressure	2–3 per cent lower risk for each 1 mmHg reduction of diastolic BP
Reducing blood cholesterol levels through exercise, diet or medication	2–3 per cent lower risk for each 1 per cent reduction in HDL cholesterol
Taking prophylactic aspirin	33 per cent lower risk in users compared with non-users

The Benefits of Aspirin

Aspirin is a commonly used pain killer and anti-inflammatory drug that also has a powerful blood thinning effect. It lowers the stickiness of platelet particles in the blood so that they are less likely to clump together and form unwanted clots. This effect occurs at only a quarter of the dose needed to relieve pain. Although there is not yet felt to be enough evidence to recommend that everyone takes prophylactic aspirin, it is often recommended for those with risk factors of coronary heart disease. Studies suggest that prophylactic aspirin can reduce the risk of a first heart attack by 33 per cent in men – there is no equivalent data on its effects in women, but it is likely to be similar. Unfortunately, taking aspirin can produce side-effects of gastric irritation, and in some people can lead to peptic ulceration and intestinal bleeding. It is therefore not suitable for everyone and should only be taken under medical supervision.

The best evidence for an alternative anti-clotting supplement is for extracts of the French maritime pine, known as pycnogenol. Its antioxidant action is 50 times more powerful than vitamin E and 20 times more powerful than vitamin C. Pycnogenol strengthens fragile capillaries and helps to protect against hardening and furring of the arteries – even in smokers. Research suggests 125 mg pycnogenol is as effective in preventing increased susceptibility to blood clotting as 500 mg aspirin, but with the advantage of not irritating the stomach and causing gastric side-effects as aspirin can. Garlic is also beneficial in reducing blood clotting (see page 175).

Stroke

A stroke is a sudden loss of control of one or more body functions due to interruption of the blood supply to part of the brain resulting in death of some brain cells (neurones). There are three main types of stroke:

- *a clot (thrombosis) in a brain artery* which cuts off the supply of oxygen-rich blood to a group of brain cells
- *a clot that forms elsewhere in the circulation* (e.g. in a carotid artery in the neck) may break off and travel in the blood-stream to the brain, where it lodges in a blood vessel to suddenly cut off the blood supply
- *haemorrhage into the brain* due to a ruptured blood vessel.

Most types of stroke are due to a combination of hypertension, atherosclerosis and increased stickiness of the blood, all of which become increasingly common in women after the menopause, when the beneficial effects of oestrogen on the circulation are lost.

Transient Ischaemic Attacks

A transient ischaemic attack (TIA) is similar to a mini-stroke, but symptoms resolve fully within 24 hours. TIAs are often recurrent and due to small platelet clumps lodging in small blood vessels within the brain to temporarily block the circulation to some brain cells. The platelet clots break up and clear before brain cells die from lack of blood. TIAs are more common after the menopause, due to the adverse effects of oestrogen withdrawal. A TIA is an important warning sign that a stroke may occur in the future – five years on from the TIA, 1 in 6 sufferers will have suffered a stroke, and 1 in 4 will have died, usually from a heart attack or stroke. If TIAs are treated by taking a drug that lowers platelet stickiness (e.g. aspirin or the natural alternative, pycnogenol – see page 82) a full-blown stroke can often be prevented

---

To help avoid a stroke

- Stop smoking
- Lose excess weight
- Exercise regularly
- Keep alcohol intake within the recommended safe amounts
- Take steps to lower raised blood fat levels
- If diabetic, make sure your blood sugar levels are always well controlled
- If you have high blood pressure, ensure it is well controlled
- Ensure a good intake of vitamin C – those with the highest intakes of vitamin C are half as likely to suffer a stroke as those with intakes of less than 28mg vitamins C per day
- Ensure a good intake of folic acid to help counter raised homocysteine levels (see page 72)
- Taking low-dose aspirin (75–150 mg) per day can reduce the risk of a heart attack or stroke by 30 per cent, and the risk of dying from them by 15 per cent. Seek medical advice before starting it, however, to ensure it is likely to suit you.

Cardiac Syndrome X

Researchers have identified a problem that mainly affects menopausal women, and which has been called Cardiac Syndrome X. It is diagnosed if:

- someone experiences typical tight angina heart pain brought on by exercise
- and, when the patient is wired up to a heart monitor and

exercised on a treadmill, the tracing shows that the heart muscle is lacking in oxygen
- but when the width of the coronary arteries is assessed using a special x-ray dye-test (angiography) no narrowing or blockages are found.

Further testing also rules out coronary artery spasm, high blood pressure, heart valve problems and other possible causes, which could possibly affect oxygen supply to the heart muscle.

At first, the cause of Cardiac Syndrome X was unknown. Then it was noticed that most patients affected were women, particularly postmenopausal women, with symptoms of oestrogen withdrawal such as hot flushes, night sweats and headache. For example, out of 134 patients in one study, 27 were male and 104 were female with an average age of 53.8 years. It also seems that women who have undergone hysterectomy are more prone to the condition.

Researchers now believe that Cardiac Syndrome X is due to a hormone imbalance which affects the way small blood vessels (capillaries) in the heart muscle react during exercise. Usually, they dilate to bring blood flooding into the exercising muscle. In Cardiac Syndrome X, it is thought that these vessels fail to dilate during exercise, so that the heart is starved of the increased amount of oxygen it needs. As a result, heart pain (angina) occurs even though the coronary arteries are perfectly healthy.

While Cardiac Syndrome X does not seem to be dangerous, in that it does not increase the risk of premature death, it does play havoc with lives as some people are so intolerant of exercise they are virtually confined to their homes. Early studies show that giving oestrogen replacement therapy can help to cut down the number of angina attacks experienced and relieve day-to-day symptoms.

Metabolic Syndrome X

One in five people are believed to suffer from Metabolic Syndrome X which is linked with a diet high in sugar and refined carbohydrates, little or no exercise, obesity and high blood pressure. Women who are post menopausal are especially at risk.

Metabolic Syndrome X is present when two or more of the following six factors are present:

- insulin resistance
- glucose intolerance
- high insulin levels
- high triglyceride levels
- low levels of beneficial HDL-cholesterol
- high blood pressure.

The underlying cause of Metabolic Syndrome X is believed to be insulin resistance, in which body cells lose their sensitivity to insulin hormone and do not respond to it properly. This usually occurs when a diet that is too high in sugar leads to overproduction of insulin hormone. Insulin is made by special beta cells within the pancreas gland. It helps to regulate blood sugar levels by promoting the transport of glucose into liver and muscle cells, where it is used as an energy fuel. Without insulin, glucose builds up in the bloodstream and body cells do not receive enough glucose to use as fuel and must switch to emergency measures. As a result, the metabolism of carbohydrate, protein and fat becomes grossly abnormal.

When too many foods that raise blood sugar levels are eaten, more insulin is secreted to store the excess sugar in fat cells. This leads to overweight – especially around the waist, to produce the classic apple shape. If you have a waist size of more than 32 inches (37 inches for male) you are at risk of developing, and could already have, Metabolic Syndrome X. People with Metabolic Syndrome X are basically overdosing on glucose and insulin. Because insulin levels are persistently high, body cells stop responding to its effects, leading to tiredness and sugar cravings – the so-called vicious circle of Metabolic Syndrome X. People with this condition ideally need to reduce their blood sugar levels, lose weight, exercise more (just 30 minutes a day can halve your risk of Syndrome X and type 2 diabetes) and switch to a type of diet that does not cause spikes in blood sugar levels. You also need to increase your intake of antioxidants to help neutralize all the harmful metabolic free radicals produce by such an abnormal metabolism. This means eating foods with a low rather than a high glycaemic index, following a high fibre diet, eating plenty of fresh fruit and vegetables and taking antioxidant supplements.

Following a low glyaemic diet, and making changes to your lifestyle can reverse Syndrome X so insulin levels fall and your cells become sensitivets the effects of normal insulin levels again (see Chapter 8: Diet and Menopause for details).

Drink plenty of fluids and cut right back on intakes of caffeine, which can increase insulin release.

Dementia and Poor Memory

Alzheimer's disease is the most common form of dementia, the symptoms of which vary from person to person. There seems to be a link between oestrogen levels, HRT and the risk of Alzheimer's in women. The first inkling that something is wrong is usually forgetfulness and loss of memory.

Long-ago events such as those occurring in childhood are often recalled, but recent facts such as what was on television the night before cannot be remembered. It then becomes increasingly difficult to concentrate, add numbers and to find the right words to describe what you mean. Although mild versions of these symptoms are perfectly normal with increasing age, overwork and stress, it soon becomes apparent that problems are more severe in someone suffering from this condition. Mood swings and personality changes occur and eventually, a person with Alzheimer's becomes very disorientated and confused.

Alzheimer's is associated with changes in the brain in which beta-amyloid plaques and proteinaceous tangles develop in brain tissues. There are oestrogen receptors in the brain and, interestingly, women taking oestrogen hormone replacement therapy for at least one year after the menopause are less likely to develop Alzheimer's disease than those who do not. Women who take oestrogen for ten years or more seem to be 30 per cent less likely to develop the condition – and if it does occur, it tends to start later than usual. Recent research also shows that someone with untreated raised blood pressure at the age of 70 is more likely to develop dementia within the next 15 years than a 70-year-old with normal BP – this applies to all forms of dementia, including Alzheimer's disease. Why Alzheimer's disease is linked with high blood pressure is not yet understood, but it is probably due to raised homocysteine levels, increased risk of atherosclerosis and poor blood supply to the brain.

It seems that maintaining an active interest in life, and using your brain to work out puzzles, crosswords etc., seems to stimulate brain cells so they are more likely to retain their connections with other brain cells, rather than withering away and dying.

Improving Your Memory

Your memory is a personal storehouse of information, including learned facts and emotional events. As you get older, it is natural for your memory to become less like a filing cabinet and more like a sieve – facts get harder to store and retrieve. There are three main types of memory:

- sensory memory briefly remembers facts for a split second
- short-term memory stores facts for around 5 minutes
- long-term memory can store facts for as long as a lifetime

How Good is Your Memory?

The most common memory problem is the mild forgetfulness that occurs with increasing age. This is sometimes known as benign senile forgetfulness and is entirely normal. Consider the following questions to assess your current memory.

SHORT-TERM MEMORY

- Do you forget whether you've locked the door or turned off the oven?
- Do you walk into a room and forget why you're there?
- Do you start a sentence then forget what you wanted to say?
- Do you read something, forget what it said and have to read it again?
- Do you keep repeating yourself?
- What did you have for breakfast?

MEDIUM-TERM MEMORY

- Can you remember what you did last weekend?
- Do you start telling a joke, then forget the punchline?
- Do you get lost on a journey you've made before?
- Do you forget to pick up the dry-cleaning or buy an item you need for supper?
- Do you plan to watch a TV programme then forget it's on?

LONG-TERM MEMORY

- Can you remember what you were doing when you heard that President Kennedy was shot/ Elvis died/Margaret Thatcher resigned?
- Can you remember your last address and post code?
- When was your first kiss, and with whom?
- Who was Prime Minister when you voted for the first time?

What is your Short-term Memory Span?

Ask someone to read the following numbers out loud to you, one at a time. After each line, try to repeat the numbers digit for digit. Continue line by line until you come to a number you cannot repeat from memory. The most number of digits you can remember correctly is your memory's digit span. For most people, this is around seven.

3
56
865
7319

34721
948735
3583827
43672181
972565647
1726834956
53749427312

Lifestyle Changes to Boost Your Memory

- Eat a healthy, wholefood diet with plenty of fresh fruit, vegetables, cereals and fish – avoid processed foods containing additives as much as possible.
- If you smoke, try to stop
- Cut back on alcohol intake
- Increase the amount of exercise you take to boost circulation to the brain
- Make sure you get enough relaxation, rest and sleep

Tips to Boost Your Memory

1. Write yourself a memory-jogging note of things to do on a piece of paper and stick it up where you will easily see it.
2. The more you stretch your brain, the better your memory. Keep your brain cells active by reading demanding books, doing crosswords and other puzzles that need concentration. Games such as Scrabble or Trivial Pursuits are excellent for testing your memory skills.
3. If you can't remember someone's name, try to remember where you met them, what they were wearing, any unusual physical characteristic or mannerism and what you talked about – this will often jog your memory.

4. If you keep losing something (e.g. your keys) try to form a mental photograph of where they are every time you put them down.

Supplements that can help to improve your memory

A number of supplements can help to improve memory. You can try the following:

- folic acid and Vitamin B12
- thiamine
- lecithin
- garlic
- ginko.

FOLIC ACID AND VITAMIN B12

Low blood levels of folic acid and vitamin B12 have been linked with an increased risk of dementia, especially Alzheimer's disease. This is thought to result from elevated blood level of the amino acid, homocysteine. Normally, homocysteine levels are tightly controlled by three enzymes that convert homocysteine to cysteine – a safe end product used by cells for growth. Two of the three enzymes that control homocysteine levels depend on folic acid for their activity. Many people do not obtain enough dietary folic acid for optimal enzyme function, or have genetic mutations that decrease the activity of these controlling enzymes. As a result, homocysteine accumulates in the circulation, causing oxidation damage to the lining of artery walls so they become narrow and inelastic. This increases the risk of coronary heart disease, stroke and dementia.

One study found those with homocysteine levels in the top third of the range were 4.5 times more likely to have

AD than those with homocysteine levels in the bottom third. A three-year follow up study also found that those with the highest homocysteine levels were more likely to show radiological evidence of greater disease progression. Increased intakes of folic acid may help to protect older people against vascular disease and preserve cognitive function. Research suggests that taking as little as 300 mcg folic acid daily is effective in lowering plasma homocysteine levels.

Thiamine

Faulty memory is occasionally due to thiamine (vitamin B1) deficiency, especially in people who drink a lot of alcohol. This is treated with high doses of around 50 mg vitamin B1 per day. Foods rich in thiamine include: brewer's yeast, brown rice, wheat germ, wholegrain bread and cereals.

Multivitamins and Minerals

Taking a good multinutrient supplement each day will act as a safety net against lack of a vitamin or mineral that may affect your memory and general health. As well as thiamine, other B group vitamins and the minerals potassium, magnesium, calcium, iron and zinc are vitally important for good memory function.

When to Seek Help

If memory loss is accompanied by confusion, poor concentration or a change in behaviour or personality, it is important to seek medical advice.

7

Osteoporosis and the Menopause

Osteoporosis is one of the most common long-term conditions to affect post-menopausal women. By the age of 60 years, 25 per cent of women have brittle bones, and by the age of 70, 50 per cent of women are affected. On average, one in four women develop an osteoporotic fracture during their life compared with only one in 40 men. This is because men start off with thicker, stronger bones, which therefore take longer to thin down enough to become brittle. Osteoporosis has reached almost epidemic proportions in the Western world, yet it is largely a preventable disease.

As with heart disease, women are relatively protected against osteoporosis until they reach the menopause. This is because the female hormone, oestrogen, acts on bone to increase its mineral content. Once oestrogen levels fall after the menopause, bone thinning naturally occurs, although hormone replacement therapy helps to prevent this.

What is Osteoporosis?

Bone is a living tissue containing a network of collagen fibres filled with calcium salts. Bone is constantly remodelling itself, with as much as 10 per cent of its mass broken down and rebuilt each year – your entire skeleton is replaced every seven to ten years. This remodelling process involves special cells (osteoclasts) dissolving old bone, while other cells (osteoblasts) lay down new bone.

The osteocytes and osteoblasts put out fine finger-like processes that interconnect and communicate with each another. This network seems to be sensitive to the everyday stresses and strains on each bone and can tell exactly where a bone needs building up. Researchers do not know exactly how the process of bone remodelling is started and stopped, although various hormones and growth factors are known to be involved.

Osteoporosis develops when the balance between bone production and bone absorption is lost so that the amount of both collagen fibres and calcium salts fall significantly. This makes bones thin and brittle so they fracture more easily. Osteoporotic bones may have so few minerals in them that they show up as pale ghosts on X-ray, rather than as strong white shadows.

Up until your mid-thirties, your bones continue to build in strength until they reach their peak density at around 35 years of age. After the menopause when oestrogen stimulation of bone formation is lost, bone thinning slowly occurs as part of a natural process. This process can be offset, however, by taking active dietary and lifestyle measures throughout life so that your bones are as strong as possible before the menopause occurs. A woman with a low bone mass at the time she reaches the menopause, has two to three times the risk of a future fracture.

The rate at which bone is lost is also important. Bone density is lost most rapidly in the ten years after the menopause, once oestrogen levels fall. The average post-menopausal woman loses 2 to 3 per cent of her bone mass each year, but some lose up to 5 per cent. By the age of 70, untreated women will lose up to 30 per cent of their pre-menopausal bone mass and a few lose a staggering 50 per cent.

What are the Symptoms of Osteoporosis?

Osteoporosis is described as the silent epidemic, for there are few symptoms or signs, even when the disease is advanced. Unfortunately, the first indication that you have a problem is often when a fracture occurs after a minor fall. Fractures of bones in the spinal column (vertebrae) can occur spontaneously or result from minor strains occurring when lifting or even coughing. These vertebral fractures are usually painful and can lead to a stooped posture and loss of height. In women, the pronounced spinal curvature is sometimes referred to as Dowager's hump.

Early osteoporosis may also cause back pain – at least in men. Spanish rheumatologists looked at 81 men with osteoporosis (average age 55) and found that in 85 per cent of cases, back pain was the first symptom. Of these, 65 per cent suffered from long-term back pain. In half the cases, this was due to a previous vertebral fracture, but most men also had a history of back pain not due to fracture. It is likely that these findings also apply to women.

Who gets osteoporosis?

Menopausal women who are at most risk of osteoporosis are those who:

- enter the menopause early, before the age of 45 – especially if this was due to hysterectomy and surgical removal of the ovaries – and who have not taken hormone replacement therapy
- have a strong family history of the disease
- have taken prolonged courses of oral corticosteroids for three months or longer
- Loss of periods for any cause except pregnancy (e.g. excessive dieting, excessive exercise, use of depot progestogen contraception)
- are underweight
- have suffered from anorexia or bulimia nervosa in the past
- have eaten a calcium-poor diet (e.g. women on a continual slimming diet, or who eat few dairy products)
- smoke or drink heavily
- take little exercise, which helps to build up bone strength
- or conversely, have exercised excessively (e.g. marathon runners; ballet dancers; exercise trainers)
- have a history of prolonged bed rest, especially in childhood
- have been bedridden for long periods of time
- have had long episodes without periods (e.g. due to hormone imbalances or, possibly, to the contraceptive injection)
- are housebound, with little exposure to sunlight and low dietary intakes of vitamin D and calcium
- have liver disease
- have overactive parathyroid glands (hyperparathyroidism).

How Osteoporosis is Diagnosed

Osteoporosis may not be diagnosed until you have an X-ray to investigate a fracture after a minor fall. If the condition is suspected, however, you may be offered bone mineral density screening to assess the strength of your bones.

The best way to identify early osteoporosis is a test known as dual energy X-ray absorbtiometry (DEXA). Private screening clinics often offer a different type of test known as quantitative ultrasound (QUS), which is used to assess future fracture risk in women who are going through or have gone through the menopause. Clinical studies show that in older women aged 70-plus, QUS can predict hip fracture risk as well as DEXA, and that it can predict wrist fracture risk in early post menopausal women. There are currently no accepted criteria for using QUS to diagnose osteoporosis, however. The National Osteoporosis Society (see Useful Addresses) has raised concerns that QUS may be used inappropriately for routine screening of young people, and that some units are staffed by inexperienced operators who are unable to perform the test, or interpret the results, properly. The NOS are aware of several people who have paid for QUS and been told they have osteoporosis, yet after having a DEXA scan they have found that they do not. If you are at risk of osteoporosis, it is best to consult your doctor, who can refer you for screening at your local hospital if appropriate.

Bone density screening cannot accurately predict who will go on to have a fracture in later life if not treated and those who won't. Two thirds of fractures occur in women with bone densities above the lowest 20 per cent which limits the effectiveness of global screening. As osteoporosis is a preventable disease, is it important to take steps as early as possible to safeguard your bones.

Preventing Osteoporosis

Osteoporosis is largely a preventable disease. Diet and lifestyle are so important to hormone balance, that stopping smoking and improving nutrition can delay the menopause by as much as three or four years. It can also delay, minimize or even prevent the onset of osteoporosis. Women who do not smoke and who keep their alcohol intake to within recommended limits by the time they reach the menopause are 40 per cent less likely to have a future hip fracture than a woman who smokes and drinks alcohol to excess. It is never too late – or too early – to take steps to reduce your risk.

Minimizing the risk of osteoporosis

- Follow a bone-friendly diet
- Obtain adequate supplies of calcium
- Get sufficient vitamin D (from diet and exposure to sunlight)
- Obtain enough of other vital vitamins and minerals important for bone health
- Take regular exercise
- Stop smoking
- Avoid excessive intake of alcohol
- Maintain your fitness, balance, alertness and eyesight as you get older to reduce the risk of falls
- Use walking aids when necessary, thinking ahead about safety in the home
- Avoid medications that may lead to confusion, dizziness or falls.

Alcohol

A moderate intake of alcohol – especially red wine – can be beneficial for health generally by reducing stress levels and lowering your risk of high blood pressure, coronary heart disease and stroke. Moderate intakes also seem to be beneficial for female bones. Post-menopausal women who drink three glasses of wine a day (or two drinks of hard liquor or three beers) seem to have a bone density that is 5–10 per cent greater than for non-drinkers, regardless of age, weight, height, smoking habits or whether they took hormone replacement therapy. Researchers have suggested that this intake of alcohol may improve bone mineral density by increasing oestrogen levels in women. The opposite effect occurs in men, however, as alcohol also lowers male testosterone levels.

Excess alcohol intake is harmful to bones, as it inhibits absorption of bone-building nutrients such as vitamin C, folic acid, calcium, copper, magnesium and zinc, affects vitamin D metabolism and increases excretion of calcium from the body. It also has a direct toxic effect against bone cells. You can help to prevent brittle bones by ensuring your intake is within the recommended safe maximum (no more than 2–3 units per day for women). Women who stop smoking and drinking at the time of the menopause may reduce their risk of a fracture by as much as 40 per cent.

Smoking

Smoking cigarettes significantly increases your risk of osteoporosis by lowering blood oestrogen levels and reducing the activity of bone-building cells (osteoblasts) so less new bone is made. Research suggests that one in eight hip fractures in women is due to smoking. For women aged 60, smokers are 17 per cent more likely than smokers to suffer a hip fracture; at 70 years, smokers are 41 per cent more likely to have a hip fracture; at 80 years, smokers are 71 per cent more likely to have a hip fracture. For tips on how to stop smoking, see pages 216–8.

Natural Plant Oestrogens

Many plants contain natural chemicals that have a weak, hormone-like action in the human body. These plant hormones, known as phytoestrogens, help to maintain falling hormone levels after the menopause and protect against osteoporosis as well as improving menopausal symptoms. For more information, see Isoflavones, page 183.

In Chapter 8, Diet and the Menopause, you will find detailed dietary recommendations for preventing and alleviating osteoporosis. Calcium plays a particularly important role here.

Osteoporosis and HRT

By replenishing your falling oestrogen levels, hormone replacement therapy boosts formation of new bone and can prevent the rapid bone loss seen in the ten years after the menopause. This protective effect continues for some years after HRT is stopped, but is not maintained indefinitely. For current users of HRT:

- risk of hip fracture is reduced by 10–40 per cent with seven or more years of use
- risk of hip fracture is reduced by 50 per cent with more than 10 years use
- In women with established osteoporosis, HRT can slow further bone loss and reduce the risk of a fracture by up to 40 per cent.

Interestingly, HRT seems to reduce the risk of an osteoporotic fracture more than would be expected from its effects on bone mass density alone. It may have other actions and increase the quality of new bone being made, as well as decreasing bone turnover.

An exciting new class of drug may one day eradicate osteoporosis. Called selective estrogen (US spelling) receptor modulators (SERMs) they switch on oestrogen receptors in bone arteries and the heart but switch off those present in the breast and uterine tissues. This gives all the benefits of hormone replacement therapy without increasing the risk of hormone-dependent cancers. The first drug to be discovered is still at the research stage.

For more information on HRT and SERMS, see Chapter 13.

8
Diet and the Menopause

After the menopause, lower levels of oestrogen increase the risk of a number of circulatory problems, including atherosclerosis, high blood pressure, angina, coronary heart disease and stroke. In this chapter, we take a look at the dietary and lifestyle changes you can take to help reduce their occurrence or severity.

Preventing Coronary Heart Disease (CHD) through Diet

People who follow a Mediterranean style diet (rich in olive oil and vegetables) have a 75 per cent lower risk of CHD than those eating a typical Western style diet (full of animal fats and convenience foods). The Mediterranean way of eating is thought to reduce the risk of atherosclerosis because it includes healthy types of fat such as olive oil, plus garlic, antioxidants, oily fish, red wine and is also rich in unrefined complex carbohydrates and fibre.

Dietary Fats

Dietary fats consist of a molecule of glycerol to which three fatty acid chains are attached in a sideways formation that produces a molecular shape similar to a capital E.

Fats that contain no double bonds are referred to as saturated fats. Fats containing some double bonds are known as unsaturated fats. Those with one double bond are mono-unsaturated, while those with two or more double bonds are polyunsaturated. Most dietary fats contain a blend of saturates, monounsaturates and polyunsaturates in varying proportions. In general, saturated fats tend to be solid at room temperature while monounsaturated and polyunsaturated fats tend to be oils.

Ideally, dietary fats should provide no more than 30 per cent of daily energy intakes. For women with an average energy intake of 1928 kcal per day, 30 per cent of food energy intake is equivalent to around 66 g of fat. The average woman should therefore aim to eat no more than around 66 g of fat per day. Unfortunately, surveys suggest that for the average adult, dietary fats currently provide over 40 per cent of daily calories, which is far too high. Most people would benefit from cutting back on their overall fat intake, while increasing their intake of the more beneficial types of fat. Check food labels to obtain information on the amount of fat provided by different foods and aim for those that are as low as possible

Saturated fats

Saturated (animal) fats are converted into cholesterol in the liver, and were traditionally thought of as the baddies when it came to coronary heart disease. But over a third of saturated fats in milk fat or butter – those with chain lengths of up to 10 carbon atoms and in excess of 16 – have no effect on blood cholesterol levels. Only saturated fats with carbon chains of 12, 14 and 16 have any reported effect. In particular, stearic acid (18 carbon atoms) found in milk fat, cocoa butter and meat fat also has no cholesterol raising activity.

One of the longest running studies into coronary heart disease found no link between high blood cholesterol levels and saturated fat intake. Researchers now increasingly believe that CHD is not so much linked to abnormally raised blood cholesterol levels, but to a lack of dietary antioxidants (e.g. vitamins C and E, carotenoids, selenium). This is because antioxidants help to protect circulating fats from chemical attack (oxidation), as it is only oxidized LDL cholesterol that is attacked by circulating scavenger cells and taken into artery walls, where they contribute to the hardening and furring up process.

This does not mean that a high saturated fat intake is not harmful, however – like all fats, it has a high calorie content and excess is linked with obesity and the complications, such as high blood pressure, to which this can lead. Also, if you have a family history of atherosclerosis, CHD or high blood cholesterol levels, you may have inherited genes that mean you process saturated fat less well than other people.

Ideally, saturated fats should supply no more than 10 per cent of your energy intake (around 22 g per day), which for most people means cutting back on the amount they obtain from their diet.

POLYUNSATURATED FATS
There are two main types of polyunsaturated fat in the diet:

- omega-3 PUFAs mainly derived from fish oils
- omega-6 PUFAs mainly derived from vegetable oils.

Researchers now increasingly believe that it is eating too much omega-6 polyunsaturated fatty acids (mainly found in vegetable oils) and not enough omega-3 polyunsaturated fatty acids (mainly found in fish oils) that increases your risk of atherosclerosis. This is especially true if your intake of antioxidants (e.g. vitamins C, E, betacarotene and mineral selenium) is low. Antioxidants, which are mainly found in fresh fruit and vegetables, help to protect body fats from a chemical alteration known as oxidation.

Unlike saturated fats, polyunsaturated fatty acids (PUFAs) have a molecular structure containing spare double bonds. This makes them highly reactive and more susceptible to chemical change through free radical attack (e.g. when attacked by chemicals released by macrophages).

Your body handles omega-3 and omega-6 oils in different ways: omega-3 fish oils have a thinning effect on your blood and help to reduce the risk of CHD and stroke, while omega-6 PUFAs are increasingly thought to be linked with inflammatory processes in the body, including coronary heart disease. The average Western diet currently contains a ratio of omega-6 to omega-3 fats of around 7:1, when ideally the ratio should be more balanced – eating more monounsaturated fats will help achieve this.

Monounsaturated Fats

Monounsaturated fats consist of chains of carbon atoms in which there is only one double (unsaturated) bond. Monounsaturated fats are metabolized in such a way that they lower harmful LDL cholesterol levels with no effect on HDL levels, and ideally, should supply around 12 per cent of your energy intake. For most people, this means eating more monounsaturates in place of omega-6 PUFAs; this would help reduce the risk of CHD as well as bringing the dietary ratio of omega-3s and omega-6s into a better balance. A diet high in monounsaturated fats may help to reduce your risk of atherosclerosis, high blood pressure, coronary heart disease and stroke. This is thought to explain some of the benefits of the so-called Mediterranean diet. Foods rich in monounsaturates include olive oil, rapeseed oil and avocado.

TRANS-FATTY ACIDS

When polyunsaturated oils are partially hydrogenated to solidify them in the production of cooking fats and spreads (e.g. margarine) some trans-fatty acids are produced. When trans-fatty acids are incorporated into your cell membranes, they increase their rigidity and also seem to raise blood levels of harmful LDL cholesterol while lowering beneficial HDL cholesterol. Trans-fatty acids have therefore been linked with an increased risk of high blood pressure and coronary heart disease. They may also interfere with the way your body handles essential fatty acids, so their beneficial effects are not fully realized.

The average consumption of dietary trans-fatty acids is around 5–7 g per day. Some people eat as much as 25–30 g of trans-fatty acids daily, particularly if they use cheap margarines and lots of processed foods. Concern about their safety is great enough that some margarines and low fat spreads have been reformulated to reduce their trans-fat content. Some countries have also introduced guidelines aimed at reducing intakes of trans fatty acids to no more than 2 per cent of your total energy intake.

Plant Sterols and Stanols

Plant sterols and stanols, substances found in virtually all plants, have a similar chemical structure to animal cholesterol. They therefore interact with the mechanisms designed to absorb pre-formed cholesterol from the diet so that less cholesterol is absorbed overall. Consuming 2 g plant sterols or stanols per day can significantly lower LDL cholesterol and help to protect against heart disease.

A number of functional foods have now been developed that are fortified with these cholesterol-lowering substances, including spreads and yoghurts. When included in a healthy diet, they help to lower LDL cholesterol by up to 15 per cent within as little as three weeks. Consuming 20–25 g of spread containing plant sterols daily can lower LDL cholesterol by 10–15 per cent.

How to reduce your risk of atherosclerosis, CHD and stroke:

- Reduce your overall consumption of fat, especially saturated fats
- Eat more monounsaturated fats (e.g. olive or rapeseed oils)
- Increase your intake of omega-3 fatty acids (mainly found in fish oils)
- Include foods fortified with plant sterols/stanols in your diet
- Reduce your intake of omega-6 fatty acids (mainly found in vegetable oils)
- Eat as few processed foods as possible to reduce your intake of trans-fatty acids and hidden fats
- Increase your intake of antioxidants (found in fruit, vegetables and supplements).

How to Cut Down on Fat

The simplest way to cut back on dietary fats is to avoid obviously fatty foods, such as doughnuts, chips, crisps and, chocolate as much as possible, and to choose reduced fat versions of foods such as dairy foods which provide other important nutrients such as calcium. Thy the following tips:

- Obtain at least half your daily calories from complex carbohydrates such as wholegrain bread, wholemeal pasta, brown rice, cereals etc. – but don't smother them in calorific sauces or spreads
- steam, boil, dry bake or poach food rather than deep frying
- grill food rather than frying to help drain fat away. Use only a light brushing of olive or rapeseed oil if necessary, plus herbs, lemon juices and spices for flavour
- dry (stir) frying using a light brushing of monounsaturated fats (e.g. olive or rapeseed oil).
- if roasting meat, place the meat on a rack within the roasting pan so fats drain away. Roast potatoes with just a light brushing of olive oil
- use skimmed or semi-skimmed rather than whole milk products
- replace butter and cream with monounsaturated products derived from olive oil or rapeseed oil
- use low-fat versions of as many foods as possible (e.g. mayonnaise, yoghurts, salad dressings, reduced fat cheese, reduced fat monounsaturated spreads, etc.)
- avoid foods high in saturated fat such as creamy soups, chocolate, pâté, oysters, prawns
- decrease the amount of red meat you eat to only once or twice per week. Have more vegetarian meals instead, which include pulses and beans for protein
- trim all visible fat from meat. Buy lean cuts
- eat more fish – preferably organic to reduce intakes of pollutants
- eat boiled or baked potatoes rather than roasted or chipped (but see Glycemic Index page 158).

Dietary factors Beneficial for the Cardiovascular System

A number of dietary components have a beneficial effect on heart and circulatory health.

OLIVE OIL

Olive oil is one of the healthiest dietary oils as it has beneficial effects on blood lipid levels. It is rich in a type of fat (oleic acid) that is monounsaturated (see pages 106–7). Oleic acid reduces absorption of cholesterol, and is processed in the body to lower the harmful LDL cholesterol without modifying desirable HDL cholesterol. It also reduces abnormal blood clotting tendencies and, as a result, in regions where olive oil is used liberally, the incidence of coronary heart disease, high blood pressure, peripheral vascular disease, stroke and other cholesterol-related illnesses – including dementia – is low. Oleic acid also has beneficial effects on insulin levels and diabetes.

A diet rich in olive oil (34 per cent total fat, with 21 per cent as monounsaturated fatty acid and only 7 per cent as saturated fat) has been shown to reduce the risk of coronary heart disease by 25 per cent. In a study involving 605 people recovering from a heart attack, those following such a diet were 56 per cent less likely to have another heart attack, or to die from heart problems, than those following their normal diet.

Among people with high blood pressure, using 30 to 40 g olive oil for cooking every day has been shown to reduce their need for anti-hypertensive drugs by almost 50 per cent over a six-month period, compared with only 4 per cent for those randomized to use sunflower oil. All those on the sunflower oil diet continued to need their anti-hypertensive drug treatment, while 80 per cent of those using olive oil were able to discontinue their drug treatment altogether. This effect was thought to be related to the antioxidant polyphenols in olive oil.

The ideal intake appears to be at least 10 g daily, and preferably 30 to 40 g daily.

GARLIC

Garlic (*Allium sativum*) is a popular kitchen herb. The main beneficial substance derived from garlic is allicin, which gives a crushed clove its characteristic smell. Allicin is present in whole garlic cloves as an odourless precursor called alliin. When garlic is crushed or sliced, alliin comes into contact with a garlic enzyme, alliinase, which breaks it down into the powerful smelling, beneficial allicin. Allicin prevents cells from taking up cholesterol, reduces cholesterol production in the liver and hastens excretion of fatty acids, to discourage atherosclerosis. Sulphur compounds formed by the degradation of allicin also act as antioxidants to protect LDL cholesterol molecules in the blood from oxidation, reducing their uptake by scavenger cells to protect against atherosclerosis.

Research shows that garlic can:

- reduce systolic BP by an average of 8 per cent and up to 16 per cent with a minimum of two to three months treatment
- lower blood pressure enough to reduce the risk of a stroke by up to 40 per cent
- reduce the risk of CHD by up to 38 per cent
- lower harmful LDL cholesterol by 12 per cent after four months treatment
- lower triglycerides by 13 per cent

- improve circulation by 48 per cent especially through small blood vessels (e.g. in the skin)
- lower the risk of blood clots by decreasing blood stickiness and platelet clumping
- hasten breakdown of any clots that do form
- help to prevent dangerous heart rhythms
- increase the fluidity of blood
- help to maintain the elasticity of important blood vessels
- promote blood vessel dilation within five hours of taking a single dose, with effects wearing off over 24 hours.

A recent study followed 152 patients for over four years and found that garlic tablets could reduce and even reverse atherosclerosis. In those not taking garlic tablets, atherosclerotic plaques built up by 15.6 per cent over the four years, while in those taking garlic, plaque volume decreased by 2.6 per cent – a combined difference of 18.2 per cent. Due to all these beneficial effects on the circulation, taking garlic extracts is estimated to reduce the risk of a heart attack by 50 per cent. It has such a powerful medicinal action that in Germany, garlic powder tablets containing the equivalent of 4 g of fresh cloves are available on prescription to treat high blood cholesterol levels and high blood pressure.

When taking garlic supplements, select a product supplying a standardized amount of allicin (1000 to 1500 mcg allicin) daily.

FISH OILS
Fish features regularly in the diets of the healthiest peoples in the world – especially those with the lowest risk of coronary heart disease, such as people eating Mediterranean and Eskimo diets. Oily fish such as salmon, trout, mackerel, salmon and sardines contain an essential fatty acid known

as EPA (eicosapentanoic acid), originally derived from algae eaten throughout the fish's life. This is processed in your body to reduce blood stickiness, platelet clumping and the formation of unwanted blood clots.

Eating fish two or three times per week has been shown to reduce the risk of heart attack and stroke. In fact, eating oily fish at least twice a week can lower your risk of CHD more than following a low-fat, high-fibre diet. Research also shows that the protective effects of oily fish are seen after only six months and after two years, those on a high fish diet are almost a third less likely to die from CHD than those not eating much fish.

Yet at the same time, it has also been suggested that oily fish should be restricted to one portion per week because of the risk of pollutants such as heavy metals, dioxins and poly-chlorinated biphenyls (PCBs). Some fish is classed as organic as it has been raised in unpolluted waters, so select these where possible. Another option is to take omega-3 fish oil supplements that have been screened for levels of pollutants. If buying fish oil capsules, choose preparations fortified with vitamin E.

Only take fish oil supplements under medical supervision if you:

- Have a tendency to easy bleeding, or are taking a blood thinning agent such as warfarin
- Are diabetic – monitor blood glucose levels carefully as control may change.

FRUIT AND VEGETABLES

Fruit, vegetables, seeds and pulses are rich sources of vita-mins, minerals – including potassium – fibre (which has beneficial effects on cholesterol absorption) plus powerful antioxidants such as vitamins C, E, carotenoids and flavonoids. Those who eat the most raw and fresh fruit have the lowest risk of developing coronary heart disease and other circulatory illnesses.

Antioxidants Antioxidants help to protect artery linings and circulating cholesterol from oxidation. Oxidation is a side-effect of harmful free radicals produced during metabolism. These damage artery linings and circulating fats, which hastens the process of atherosclerosis. Dietary antioxidants help to neutralize these free radicals before they can do any damage. The most important dietary antioxidants are vitamins C, E, carotenoids and the mineral selenium, which are found in fruit and vegetables.

The risk of developing angina and CHD is up to three times lower in people with high blood levels of vitamins E, C and carotenoids. Those who have a high intake of vitamin C (including the use of supplements) have up to a 40 per cent lower risk of CHD and a 35 per cent less risk of dying from it. Those with the highest intakes of vitamin E have up to a 75 per cent lower risk of CHD, while women with the highest intakes of carotenoids have over a 22 per cent lower risk of CHD.

Good dietary sources of carotenoids include dark green leafy vegetables and yellow-orange fruits such as:

- carrots, sweet potatoes
- spinach, broccoli, watercress, spring greens
- cantaloupe melons, apricots, peaches, mango
- red-yellow peppers
- tomatoes
- sweetcorn.

Good dietary sources of vitamin C include:

- citrus fruit
- blackcurrants, strawberries
- kiwi fruit
- guavas, mangoes
- green peppers
- green sprouting vegetables (e.g. broccoli, sprouts, watercress, parsley)

Good dietary sources of vitamin E include:

- wheatgerm oil
- avocado pear
- wholemeal cereals
- seeds
- nuts
- oily fish
- broccoli.

Flavonoids are also beneficial. These natural antioxidants help to protect cell membranes from damage to help prevent hardening and furring up of the arteries. Almost every fruit and vegetables contains flavonoids, of which over 20,000 are known to exist. One study found that men who ate the most flavonoids had less than half the number of fatal heart attacks compared with those who ate the least. The chief sources of flavonoids in the study were apples, onions and tea.

Servings The benefits of eating more fruit and vegetables – at least five servings per day, and preferably eight to ten – are so great that some experts now recommend increased intakes of antioxidants from fruit, vegetables, green and black tea and red wine (in moderation), rather than advocating a low-cholesterol, low-saturated-fat diet. A serving or portion of fruit and vegetables is basically the amount you are happy to eat in one sitting – the more the better. Typically, this would amount to:

- a glass of fruit juice
- a large mixed salad
- one large beef tomato or two medium tomatoes
- a handful of grapes, cherries or berries
- a single apple, orange, kiwi, peach, pear, nectarine or banana
- ½ grapefruit, ½ ogen melon, ½ mango, ½ papaya
- two to four dates, figs, satsumas, passion fruit, apricots, plums or prunes
- a handful of nuts
- a generous helping of green or root vegetables (excluding potatoes).

FIBRE

Eating the equivalent of 30 g fibre per day will decrease your risk of CHD by absorbing dietary fats in the gut. These means they reach your blood stream more slowly, so that your body can handle them more easily. The most beneficial type of fibre seems to be soluble oat fibre – just 3 g per day (roughly equivalent to two large bowls of porridge) can lower total blood cholesterol levels by up to 0.16 mmol. This is a small but significant change.

WALNUTS

Walnuts contain a high ratio of monounsaturated and

polyunsaturated to saturated fats. Compared to most other nuts, which contain monounsaturated fatty acids, walnuts are unique because they are rich in omega-6 (linoleic) and omega-3 (linolenic) polyunsaturated fatty acids.

A recent analysis of five clinical trials involving around 200 people consistently found that walnuts lower blood cholesterol concentrations when included in a heart-friendly diet. Studies using almonds and hazelnuts have also revealed beneficial effects on blood lipid profiles. Researchers have found that adding 84 g walnuts to the diet every day for four weeks reduced total blood cholesterol level by 12 per cent more than a control group not eating walnuts. Even more importantly, harmful LDL cholesterol levels were reduced by 16 per cent.

It is best to buy walnuts in shells or vacuum packs, as exposure to air rapidly reduces their nutrient value. Most people eat less than 4 g walnuts per week. Increasing your intake to 28 g per day would help to decrease blood LDL cholesterol levels by 6 per cent Although walnuts are energy rich (60 g supplies 578 kcals) dietary intervention studies show that eating walnuts does not cause a net gain in body weight when they are eaten as a replacement food.

TEA

Tea is one of the most popular drinks in the world. Green and black tea are similar, in that both are made from the young leaves of the same shrub, *Camellia sinensis*. Green tea is made by steaming and drying fresh tea leaves immediately after harvesting, while black tea is made by crushing and fermenting freshly cut tea leaves so they oxidize before drying. This allows natural enzymes in the tea leaves to produce the characteristic red-brown colour and reduced astringency.

Over 30 per cent of the dry weight of green tea leaves consists of powerful flavonoid antioxidants such as catechins. Green tea extracts have an antioxidant action at least 100 times more powerful than vitamin C, and 25 times more powerful than vitamin E. These are converted into less active antioxidants (e.g. theaflavins and thearubigins) during fermentation but drinking four to five cups of black tea per day still provides over 50 per cent of the total dietary intake of flavonoid antioxidants (other sources include fruit and vegetables especially apples and onions).

Drinking either green or black tea has beneficial effects on blood pressure, blood lipids, blood stickiness and can decrease the risk of CHD and stroke. Those drinking at least four cups of tea a day are half as likely to have a heart attack than non-tea drinkers.

BEWARE TABLE SALT

Common table salt, sodium chloride, plays an important role in cell functions, and a certain amount of sodium is essential for good health. However, research suggests that in some people, the rise in blood pressure seen with increasing age is directly linked to a lifetime's excessive intake of salt. Only around one in two people are sensitive to the effects of salt, however – there seems to be a poorly understood interaction between salt intake and other factors such as the genes you have inherited. Researchers have found, for example, that people with the highest blood levels of the kidney hormone, renin, are most likely to respond to following a low sodium, high potassium diet.

If you have high blood pressure, it is certainly worth cutting back on salt intake as the menopause approaches. Average intakes are currently around 6 g daily, but many people obtain twice this amount. It is estimated that reducing salt intake from 9 g to 6 g can lower your risk of a stroke by 22 per cent and your risk of death from CHD by 16 per cent. Studies suggest that not adding salt during cooking or at the table will lower your systolic blood pressure by at least 5 mmHg. If everyone did this, it is estimated that the incidence of stroke in the population would be reduced by as much as 26 per cent and coronary heart disease by 15 per cent.

Unfortunately, three quarters of dietary salt is hidden in processed foods, including canned products, ready-prepared meals, biscuits, cakes and breakfast cereals. This means it is important to check labels of bought products and avoid those containing high amounts of salt. When checking labels, those giving salt content as sodium need to be multiplied by 2.5 to give true salt content. For example, a serving of soup containing 0.4 g sodium contains 1 g salt.

To cut back on salt intake avoid:

- Obviously salty foods such as crisps, bacon, salted nuts
- Tinned products, especially those canned in brine
- Cured, smoked or pickled fish/meats
- Meat pastes, pâtés
- Ready-prepared meals
- Packet soups and sauces
- Stock cubes and yeast extracts.

Where salt is essential, use mineral-rich rock salt rather than table salt, or use a low-sodium brand of salt sparingly. Salt is easily replaceable with herbs and spices, as it doesn't take long to retrain your taste buds. Adding lime juice to food stimulates tastes buds and decreases the amount of salt you need, too.

POTASSIUM

Potassium is an important mineral, as it helps to flush excess sodium out of the body through the kidneys, where a mechanism exists to swap sodium and potassium ions in the walls of kidney tubules. Because the kidneys swap sodium for potassium in this way, a diet that is low in potassium is linked with a higher risk of high blood pressure and stroke – especially if your diet is also high in sodium. In one study, people taking anti-hypertensive medication were able to reduce their drug dose by half (under medical supervision) after increasing the potassium content of their food.

Ideally, you need to obtain around 3500 mg potassium per day. Most people get less than this however, as the average intake is around 3187 mg. Some people obtain as little as 1700 mg potassium from their food.

To increase your potassium intake eat more:

- Seafood
- Fresh fruit, especially bananas, dried apricots, pears and tomatoes
- Fruit juices and fruit yoghurts
- Vegetables especially mushrooms, potatoes, aubergines, peppers, squash and spinach
- Pulses such as peas and lima beans
- wholegrain breakfast cereals (check labels for sodium chloride content)

Steam rather than boil vegetables to retain more of their mineral content. In general, fresh wholefoods are a good source of potassium and contain little sodium (e.g. freshly squeezed orange juice) while processed food (e.g. orange cordial) usually have a reversed sodium:potassium ratio and contain little potassium but lots of sodium.

Low-salt products containing potassium chloride to replace sodium chloride are popular, but can taste bitter and should not be used excessively.

RED WINE

Many studies have found that a moderate intake of alcohol (20–30 g per day) reduces the risk of coronary heart disease by as much as 40 per cent. Red wine seems particularly beneficial, especially if drunk with meals.

Red wine contains many compounds with an antioxidant action. These help to neutralize the free radicals produced as a result of general metabolism, and which are thought to oxidize low density cholesterol and hasten narrowing and hardening of the arteries. The phenolic compounds found in red wine are able to inhibit the oxidation of LDL cholesterol significantly more than does vitamin E, and they also inhibit blood clotting (thrombosis), both of which help to reduce the development of atherosclerosis. Red wine also contains procyanidins at concentrations of up to 1 g/l. These polyphenols are also powerful antioxidants and free-radical scavengers.

Red wine also contains a natural antifungal agent derived from grape skins, called resveratrol. Resveratrol has been shown to help raise levels of protective HDL cholesterol as well as inhibiting platelet aggregation and clot formation in laboratory tests.

Much evidence has accumulated to suggest that moderate drinkers (two to three units of alcohol per day) have a lower blood pressure, less risk of a stroke and reduced risk of serious atherosclerosis as well as a lower incidence of coronary heart disease. In a study involving 129,000 people, drinking wine was associated with a significantly lower risk of cardiovascular death (a 30 per cent reduction for men and a 40 per cent reduction for women) when compared with spirit drinkers.

The beneficial effects of alcohol must be weighed up against the bad, however. Those who binge drink at weekends have almost twice the risk of sudden cardiovascular death, due to heart rhythm abnormalities, than moderate or non-drinkers. Heavy drinkers also have an increased risk of death from accidents and cirrhosis of the liver.

The key, therefore, is in moderation. Safe maximum alcohol intakes per week remain at no more than 2 to 3 units of alcohol per day for women (3 to 4 for men). A weekly intake of over 35 units for women (over 50 units for men) is considered dangerous.

---

1 unit of alcohol (10g alcohol) is equivalent to:

- 100 ml wine (one small glass) *or*
- 50 ml sherry (one measure) *or*
- 25 ml spirit (one tot) *or*
- 300 ml beer (½ pint).

Supplements

A number of food and herbal supplements are helpful for menopausal women at increased risk of coronary heart disease or other circulatory problems. Those covered elsewhere in this book include olive oil (see pages 110–11), omega-3 fish oils (see pages 112-13), folic acid (see page 143), isoflavones (see pages 149–50), garlic (see pages 111–2) and green tea (see pages 117–8).

Supplements discussed here include:

Vitamin C
Vitamin E
Calcium
Magnesium
Co-enzyme Q10
L-Carnitine
Hawthorn
Dandelion
Bilberry
Ginkgo
Lecithin
Flaxseed oil
Hempseed oil

VITAMIN C

Vitamin C is a dietary antioxidant that protects fluid parts of the body from harmful oxidation reactions that would damage cells and increase the process of atherosclerosis. Lack of vitamin C is now recognized as a risk factor for developing heart attack or stroke. In one study involving over 6,600 men and women, those with the highest vitamin C levels enjoyed a 27 per cent lower risk of coronary heart disease and a 26 per cent lower risk of stroke than those with low levels. Intakes of 250 mg to 1000 mg per day are recommended.

VITAMIN E

Vitamin E is a dietary antioxidant that protects fatty parts of the body from damaging oxidation reactions. This slows the progression of atherosclerosis and reduces the risk of blood clot formation. The Cambridge Heart Antioxidant

Study (CHAOS) divided around 2000 people with coronary heart disease into two groups. Half took vitamin E for 18 months, while half received inactive placebo. Taking high dose vitamin E (at least 400 i.u. daily) was found to reduce the risk of a heart attack by as much as 77 per cent. The protective effect was so strong, it seemed the group treated with vitamin E were at no greater risk of another heart attack than people who did not have coronary heart disease. Other large trials have shown you can reduce the risk of ever developing CHD by as much as 40 per cent through taking vitamin E supplements – the risk is lowest in those taking at least 100 IU (around 67 mg) vitamin E per day for at least two years.

CALCIUM

Low intakes of calcium have been linked with an increased risk of high blood pressure and stroke. Lack of calcium is thought to affect the way your circulation responds to changes in blood pressure detected by pressure receptors in blood vessel walls. Drugs that affect calcium channels in the body are highly successful in treating hypertension, angina, some irregular heart rhythms and poor circulation.

The EU recommended daily intake for calcium is 800 mg per day, although to prevent osteoporosis, some people need a daily intake of 1000–1500 g per day (see page 132). Some experts recommend that someone with high blood pressure should consider taking a 1000 mg calcium supplement (plus magnesium, see below) with their evening meal (when calcium flux in your body is greatest) for two months to see if this produces a fall in BP.

MAGNESIUM

Magnesium is essential for maintaining the electrical stability of cells. It is especially important in controlling calcium entry into heart cells to trigger a regular heart beat, and low intakes of magnesium have been linked with an increased risk of high blood pressure and stroke. Researchers have found that people with low levels of magnesium are more at risk of spasm of the coronary arteries (linked with angina or heart attack) as well as high blood pressure.

Foods containing magnesium include:

- soya beans
- nuts
- Brewer's yeast
- wholegrains
- seafood
- meat
- eggs
- dairy products
- bananas
- dark green, leafy vegetables.

Food processing removes most magnesium content, however.

If you have high BP, a supplement containing magnesium is a good idea. Intakes of 150 to 400 mg daily are recommended. These are best taken with food to optimize absorption. Magnesium citrate is most readily absorbed, while magnesium gluconate is less likely to cause intestinal side effects such as diarrhoea.

If taking magnesium supplements, ensure you also have a good intake of calcium.

CO-ENZYME Q10
Co-enzyme Q10 (CoQ10) is a vitamin-like substance needed to process oxygen in cells, and to generate energy-rich

molecules. It also acts together with vitamin E to form a powerful antioxidant defence against atherosclerosis and heart disease.

Levels of CoQ10 start to decrease over the age of 20 years, as dietary CoQ10 is absorbed less efficiently from the intestines and its production in body cells starts to fall. This is especially the case after the menopause. Lack of CoQ10 mean that cells – including heart muscle cells – do not receive all the energy they need, so they function at a sub-optimal level and are more likely to become diseased and to age prematurely. Research suggests falling CoQ10 levels play a significant role in age-related medical conditions such as coronary heart disease.

Supplements have been used to normalize high blood pressure and, in a trial involving 18 people with high blood pressure, 100 mg CoQ10 per day significantly reduced blood pressure compared with a placebo. Average systolic pressure fell by 10.6 mmHg, and diastolic pressure by 7.7 mmHg when taking CoQ10, but did not change with the placebo. CoQ10 is thought to lower hypertension by improving the elasticity and reactivity of the blood vessel wall.

Doses of 30 to 100 mg CoQ10 daily are recommended. Higher doses may be suggested to treat illnesses such as severe heart disease and high blood pressure, under medical supervision. CoQ10 is best taken with food to improve absorption as it is fat soluble.

L-CARNITINE

L-carnitine is a non-essential amino acid that acts as an antioxidant and speeds up energy production in cells. Its most important role is in regulating fat metabolism. It is needed to transport long-chain fatty acids into the energy-producing mitochondria found in all body cells where they are burned to produce energy. The more L-carnitine available, the more fat can be burned – especially in heart muscle cells. Providing additional L-carnitine may help to minimize heart damage in those at risk of a heart attack. Carnitine and co-enzyme Q10 seem to work synergistically.

Among a group of 44 men with angina, almost 23 per cent who took L-carnitine supplements for four weeks became free of exercise-induced angina, compared with only 9 per cent taking are inactive placebo. Results are likely to be similar in post-menopausal women. L-carnitine has also been shown to improve the distance walked without pain in patients with calf pain (intermittent claudication) due to atherosclerosis.

Dose: 250 mg to 1 g daily is recommended.

Note: If you have a medical disorder or are on prescription drugs, seek advice from a nutritional therapist before taking L-carnitine.

HAWTHORN

The flowering tops and berries of the hawthorn are one of the most beneficial herbal remedies available for treating the heart and circulation. Hawthorn extracts contain a substance, known as vitexin, that normalizes the cardio-vascular system, either relaxing or stimulating it as necessary, and may therefore be recommended to treat opposing problems. Hawthorn helps to relax peripheral blood vessels, improve circulation to the heart, reduce the risk of angina and normalize blood pressure. It has a mild diuretic action which discourages fluid retention, and can also slow or possibly even reverse the build-up of atheromatous plaques to reduce atherosclerosis. Hawthorn extracts also increase the strength and efficiency of the heart's pumping action. Other beneficial actions include promoting calm, reducing stress and overcoming insomnia.

For menopausal women, hawthorn tops are useful to:

- reduce heavy menstrual bleeding
- relieve hot flushes
- discourage fluid retention by boosting the circulation
- help depression or anxiety.

Dose: 100 to 450 mg daily (standardized to at least 1.8 per cent vitexin). Larger amounts are usually divided between three doses.

Note: Hawthorn extracts may take up to two months to show an appreciable effect. Side-effects are rare, although nausea, sweating and skin rashes have been reported. If you suffer from a heart condition, check with your doctor before taking it, especially if you are on prescribed medication.

DANDELION

Dandelion leaf (*Taraxacum officinalis*) has a diuretic action, helping to increase the elimination of excess water from the body. Dandelion also has a useful mineral content, including potassium, which helps to flush excess sodium through the kidneys. It can reduce fluid retention and has a mild blood pressure lowering action. Interestingly, dandelion does not seem to have a diuretic action in those with a normal healthy fluid balance who do not need to lose excess water.

Dose: 500 mg extracts twice a day.

Note: Do not use if you have active gallstones or obstructive jaundice.

BILBERRY

Bilberries (*Vaccinium myrtillus*) are a rich source of tannins, anthocyanins and flavonoid glycosides that have powerful antioxidant and anti-inflammatory properties. Extracts are widely used to strengthen blood vessels and the collagen-containing connective tissue that supports them, as well as improving circulation. In appears to reduce the risk of stroke and inhibit unwanted clot formation.

Bilberry also contains a unique anthocyanoside, myrtillin, which helps to lower a raised blood sugar level through a similar action to insulin.

Dose: Dry extract (25 per cent anthocyanosides): 80–160 mg, three times daily.

Note: Those with diabetes may be advised to take more than this.

GINKGO

Ginkgo biloba contains a variety of powerful antioxidants plus unique chemicals known as ginkgolides and bilobalides. These help to relax blood vessels in the body and boost blood circulation to the brain, hands, feet and genitals by stopping cell fragments in the blood (platelets) from clumping together. Many people find it helps to improve memory and concentration, as well as easing dizziness and improving their peripheral circulation – problems which can accompany long-standing high blood pressure and atherosclerosis.

Dose: 120 mg per day (select extracts standardized for at least 24 per cent ginkgolides).

Note: Do not take if also on warfarin, aspirin or other or other blood thinning medication.

PHOSPHATIDYL CHOLINE (LECITHIN)

Lecithin acts as an emulsifier to help break down dietary fats into smaller particles that can be absorbed and used in the body. Supplements appear to reduce the risk of CHD by inhibiting intestinal absorption of cholesterol and increasing excretion of cholesterol in bile which lowers a raised cholesterol level. When 32 people with high blood lipids took 10.5 g lecithin for 30 days, average total cholesterol and triglycerides decreased by one-third, harmful LDL cholesterol decreased by 38 per cent and beneficial HDL cholesterol increased by 46 per cent.

The usual recommended dose is 1 to 2 daily, usually divided into three doses. Higher doses are best taken under supervision of a nutritional therapist. Best taken with meals to boost absorption.

Note: Supplements should not be taken by those with manic depression, in case it makes their condition worse.

FLAXSEED OIL

Flaxseed oil (*Linum usitatissimum*) is a rich plant source of an omega-3 essential fatty acid, alpha-linolenic acid, similar to the essential fatty acids found in fish oil, but less potent. For those who are allergic to fish, or who don't like fishy burps, flaxseed oil is a good alternative. Flaxseed oils also contains a beneficial omega-6 essential fatty acid, linolenic acid.

Flaxseed oil has beneficial effects on circulating blood fats, including LDL cholesterol and is widely recommended for people with coronary heart disease and high blood pressure. Some evidence suggests that, as with fish oils, if taken by those who have had a heart attack it may reduce the chance of a second heart attack occurring.

Dose: 1 to 2 tablespoons twice a day. Best taken with food to enhance absorption.

HEMP SEED OIL (*CANNABIS SATIVA*)

Oil from the seed of the non-drug strain of Cannabis, known as the hemp plant, contains both omega-6 and omega-3 essential fatty acids in a ratio of three to one, which includes gammalinolenic acid (GLA). Hemp seed oil has similar uses to evening primrose, flaxseed and omega-3 fish oils and can help to maintain a healthy circulation.

Dose: 5 ml to 15 ml daily, best taken with food.

Bone Friendly Diet – Combating Osteoporosis

There are several ways in which your diet and nutritional state affects your hormone balance and bone health. The most important dietary links with your risk of osteoporosis are the amount of:

- natural plant hormones (phytoestrogens) present in your food
- essential fatty acids you obtain
- saturated fat you eat
- fibre you eat

- protein you eat
- vitamins, minerals and trace elements you obtain.

Calcium

Your body contains around 1.2 kg calcium stored in the skeleton, while around 10 g is dissolved in your body fluids. Ninety-nine per cent of calcium absorbed from the gut goes straight into your bones and teeth, while the other 1 per cent plays an important role in blood clotting, muscle contraction, nerve conduction, regulating metabolic enzymes, energy production and the smooth functioning of the immune system.

Dietary calcium is absorbed in your small intestine, a process that is dependent upon the presence of vitamin D. The process is not that efficient and usually only 30–40 per cent of dietary calcium is absorbed from the gut – the remainder is lost in your bowel motions.

HOW MUCH CALCIUM DO YOU NEED?

The National Osteoporosis society recommend the following daily intakes of calcium:

- women 19–45 years: 1000 mg per day
- women over 45 years   1500 mg per day.

In 1990, the average calcium intake in the UK was 820 mg per day, with 50 per cent of people obtaining less than this. Adding calcium supplements to the diet of elderly people reduces their risk of a vertebral fracture by 20 per cent, while giving them both calcium and vitamin D supplements may reduce their risk of non-vertebral and hip fracture by 30–40 per cent.

Possible signs of calcium deficiency:

- Muscle aches and pains
- Muscle twitching and spasm
- Muscle cramps
- Tetany (sustained cramps)
- Palpitations
- Receding gums
- Infected gums (periodontal disease)
- Loose teeth.

SOURCES OF CALCIUM

A balanced diet containing good supplies of calcium-rich foods is essential for maintaining strong bones and to help prevent osteoporosis. Lack of dietary calcium means that your bone stores of calcium are raided to maintain normal blood calcium levels. If this continues for any length of time, your risk of future osteoporosis is significantly increased. Good intakes of calcium are therefore vital throughout life – during childhood and adolescence when bones are still developing, as well as in later years when bones are naturally starting to thin down. Low intake of calcium has also been linked with an increased risk of high blood pressure and stroke. In fact, drugs that affect calcium channels in the body are highly successful in treating hypertension, angina, some irregular heart rhythms and poor circulation.

Dietary sources of calcium include:

- Milk (skimmed, semi-skimmed and full-fat contain the same amounts of calcium)
- Dairy products such as cheese, yoghurt, fromage frais
- Green leafy vegetables (e.g. broccoli)
- Salmon
- Nuts and seeds
- Pulses
- White and brown bread – in the UK, white and brown flour are fortified with calcium by law – but not wholemeal flour
- eggs.

Calcium content of some foods

Food	Calcium Content
Skimmed milk (600 ml)	720 mg
Semi-skimmed milk (600 ml)	720 mg
Whole milk (600 ml)	690 mg
Soya milk (600 ml)	78 mg
Whole milk yoghurt (150 ml)	300 mg
Low fat yoghurt (150 ml)	285 mg
Cheddar cheese (30 g)	216 mg
Fromage frais (30 g)	27 mg
Cottage cheese (30 g)	22 mg
2 slices white bread	76 mg
2 slices brown bread	76 mg
2 slices wholemeal bread	41 mg
1 egg	25 mg
1 large orange	58 mg

Spinach, boiled (112 g)	672 mg
Sardines (56 g)	220 mg
Brazil nuts (56 g)	101 mg
Figs, dried (28 g)	78 mg
Baked beans (112 g)	50 mg
Winter cabbage, boiled (112 g)	43 mg

FACTORS INTERFERING WITH CALCIUM ABSORPTION AND MINERALIZATION OF BONE

Heavy consumption of alcohol, coffee, meat and salt can reduce the amount of calcium you absorb from your diet and are linked with low bone mass and early osteoporosis. Safe intakes of alcohol however (no more that 2–3 units per day for women, no more than 3–4 units per day for men) may increase bone density and reduce the risk of osteoporosis, although this is still under investigation.

Long-term use of antacids containing aluminium have been shown to interfere with calcium deposition in bone and if used regularly for more than ten years, can double your risk of developing a hip fracture. Some types of dietary fibre (phytates from wheat in unleavened bread, e.g. chapatti) can bind calcium in the bowel to form an insoluble salt that you cannot absorb.

BOOSTING CALCIUM ABSORPTION FROM THE GUT

In order to process dietary calcium, you need a good supply of vitamin D. This is made in small amounts in the skin on exposure to sunlight. It is also present in fish liver oil, oily fish (e.g. sardines, mackerel, herring, tuna, salmon, pilchards) eggs, liver and fortified milk or margarine (which must contain vitamin D by law).

As well as a calcium-rich diet, a high intake of fruit and vegetables has recently been shown to protect against osteoporosis. These contain other micronutrients such as potassium, magnesium and vitamin C that are also important for bone health.

A diet rich in essential fatty acids (EFAs) seems to stimulate uptake of calcium from the gut, lower calcium loss in the urine and trigger increased laying down of calcium in your bones. The EFAs of most benefit are those found in evening primrose oil and oily fish. Good sources of EFAs include:

- sunflower and rapeseed oils
- evening primrose oil
- most nut oils (except peanut)
- dark green leafy vegetables
- oily fish – such as mackerel, herring, salmon and sardines

Many vegetables contain natural oestrogen-like plant hormones known as phytoestrogens (see Isoflavones page 149). Some researchers believe that eating these foods helps to maintain falling oestrogen levels at the menopause and protect against osteoporosis. These oestrogen-rich plants include:

- soya beans and soy products
- red clover
- green and yellow vegetables
- broccoli
- celery
- fennel
- liquorice
- rhubarb
- linseed
- ginseng

SHOULD YOU TAKE CALCIUM SUPPLEMENTS?

Ideally, as much calcium as possible should come from your diet. The easiest way to boost your intake is to drink an extra pint of skimmed or semi-skimmed milk per day, which will provide an additional 700 mg daily calcium. If you are unable to eat dairy products, however, calcium supplements are important. Some supplements contain calcium salts which are relatively insoluble and pass through the gut unabsorbed. For this reason, effervescent tablets, or those that dissolve in water to make citrus flavoured drinks, are thought to be more effective. New formulations that are sodium, potassium and colour free are also available.

Research suggests that adding calcium supplements to the diet of elderly people reduces their risk of a vertebral fracture by 20 per cent, while giving them both calcium and vitamin D supplements reduces their risk of non-vertebral and hip fracture by 30–40 per cent.

Note: People with a tendency to kidney stones should only take calcium supplements under the supervision of a doctor.

VITAMIN D

Vitamin D is essential for healthy bones and teeth as it is needed for the absorption of dietary calcium and phosphate from the small intestines.

Vitamin D can be made in the skin by the action of sunlight on a cholesterol-like molecule found in skin cells. Only ultra-violet light of a certain wavelength can trigger this reaction (290 nm – 310 nm) and this is mostly missing from British sunlight between the end of October and the end of March. Blood levels of vitamin D are therefore naturally higher in the summer and lower in winter. For the remainder of the year, these wavelengths mainly occur between 11.00 a.m. and 3.00 p.m., and are readily blocked by clouds.

Just going without sunlight exposure for six weeks – as many women do during winter months – can lower your vitamin D stores enough to reduce calcium absorption from the diet. Women who live in high altitudes, cover up their skin in sunlight or stay indoors all day are not exposed to enough sunlight to meet their vitamin D needs naturally and must therefore obtain it from their diet.

Try to get some fresh air outdoors every day – just 15 minutes exposure to bright sunshine on your face is enough to generate your vitamin D needs during summer, although you will need at least 30 minutes exposure to daylight for the same benefit during winter. Dark skinned people need more sun exposure than those who are fair-skinned to meet their vitamin D needs.

Phosphorus

Ninety per cent of the body's phosphorus stores are found in bones and teeth. Phosphorus combines with calcium to form calcium phosphate (hydroxyapatite), which is the main structural mineral in bone. Vitamin D is essential for absorption of phosphorus as well as calcium from the gut and for its deposition in bones. A balance between calcium and phosphorus is essential for bone health and too much or too little phosphorus can both lead to osteoporosis. The EU RDA is 800 mg per day, and good dietary sources include wholegrain cereals, dairy products, soy beans, nuts, meat and fish.

The current Western diet commonly contains two to four times more phosphorus than calcium, which is added to processed foods as a stabilizer, thickening agent, binder, acidulant and flavouring agent – especially in fizzy drinks such as colas. This excess can contribute to a significant thinning of bone after the menopause. It is therefore important to avoid processed foods as much as possible.

Magnesium

Magnesium is mineral now known to be important for healthy bones. It helps to regulate production of calcitonin and parathyroid hormone, which are involved in bone remodelling. It is needed to activate vitamin D so calcium can be absorbed from the gut, and for the production of bone crystals by the enzyme alkaline phosphatase. Seventy per cent of our body stores are found in bones and teeth. Good sources include seafood, meat, wholegrains, dark green, leafy vegetables, soy beans, brown rice, diary products.

Taking magnesium supplements (250–750 mg daily) for two years has been shown to increase bone mineral density by up to 8 per cent. Magnesium and calcium work closely together and if you are taking supplements of one, you should also take the other.

Vitamin K

Vitamin K is needed for the synthesis of osteocalcin – a calcium-binding protein found in bone matrix. Vitamin K is therefore as important for bone health as calcium. In one study, when vitamin K supplements were given to postmenopausal women, bone calcium loss was reduced by up to 50 per cent and their bones became stronger. There is currently no EU RDA set for vitamin K, but requirements are thought to be around 1 mcg per kilogram of body weight per day. Bacteria in the gut produce some vitamin K which can be absorbed and used. Good dietary sources include cauliflower (richest source), dark green leafy vegetables, yoghurt, egg yolk, alfalfa, safflower, rapeseed, soya and olive oils, fish liver oils, liver and meat.

Boron

Boron is a trace element mainly found in fruit and vegetables, and a relatively high boron intake (around 10 mg per day) may account for the lower risk of osteoporosis in vegetarians. Boron helps to normalize oestrogen production in post-menopausal women and boosts production of the active form of vitamin D. There is currently no EU RDA for boron, but many supplements aimed at people over the age of 50 include it in their formulation. It appears to be especially beneficial for older women, as a group of post-menopausal women who were given boron supplements (3 mg daily) were found to excrete 44 per cent less calcium and 33 per cent less magnesium within just eight days of treatment, compared to when they were following a low boron diet. In addition, they almost doubled their production of both oestrogen and testosterone hormones. Eating the recommended five servings of fruit and vegetables per day will provide between 1.5 and 3 mg of boron.

Manganese

Manganese is mineral found in bones and which is essential for production of cartilage, collagen and mucopolysaccharides, all of which are important for the repair, mineralization and remodelling of bone. There is currently no EU RDA set for manganese, but intakes of 2–5 mg per day are suggested. Good dietary sources include black tea – one cup of tea contains 1 mg manganese – whole grains, fruit, nuts, seeds, dark green leafy vegetables, shellfish and dairy products.

Women with osteoporosis have been found to have manganese levels that are four times lower than those without osteoporosis.

Copper

Copper is a trace element essential for the synthesis of collagen – the structural protein that forms the matrix on which calcium salts are laid down to form the skeleton. Copper is therefore important for maintaining healthy bones, and copper deficient diets have been shown to reduce bone strength. There is currently no EU RDA for copper, but intakes between 0.8 and 1.2 mg are suggested. Good dietary sources include shellfish, nuts, pulses, wholegrain cereals and green vegetables grown in copper-rich soil. Copper supplementation may be important in preventing osteoporosis if the diet is deficient. Interestingly, many people with arthritis have low blood levels of copper, and wearing a copper bracelet so trace amounts of the mineral are absorbed through the skin is a popular arthritis remedy.

Silicon

In its soluble (colloidal) form, silicic acid, is needed to help strengthen collagen and elastin fibres. The silica acid content of bones decreases with age and taking supplements containing silica has been found to strengthen bone by cross-linking collagen strands and improving mineralisation. There is currently no EU RDA for silicon, but intakes of 20–30 mg daily have been suggested. Dietary sources include wholegrains, dark green leafy vegetables, root vegetables, sweet peppers, nuts, seeds and supplements containing the herb horsetail (*Equisetum arvense*).

Zinc

Zinc is a mineral that enhances the actions of vitamin D, so it is essential for calcium absorption, production of bone collagen and for bone repair. Women with osteoporosis have been found to have blood and bone levels of zinc that are up to 30 per cent lower than in women with healthy bones. The EU RDA for zinc is 15 mg, and good dietary sources include seafood, red meat, whole grains, pulses, eggs and cheese.

Vitamin C

Vitamin C (ascorbic acid) is essential for the synthesis of collagen, a major structural protein that makes up 30 per cent of bone volume. Vitamin C stimulates bone-building cells (osteoblasts), enhances vitamin D activity and boosts calcium absorption from the gut. The EU RDA is 60 mg, although increasing numbers of people feel that 250–1000 mg is necessary for optimum health. Good dietary sources of vitamin C include berry fruits, citrus fruits, kiwi fruit, mangoes, green peppers and green sprouting vegetables.

Vitamin B6

Vitamin B6 (pyridoxine) is needed for the production of hydrochloric acid in the stomach so that calcium can be absorbed. It is also necessary for cross-linking collagen (bone matrix material) and for breaking down homocysteine – an amino acid which in excess is linked with osteoporosis and heart disease. Production of new bone is lower when there is a deficiency of vitamin B6, and it has been linked with osteoporosis and increased risk of hip fractures. The EU RDA for vitamin B6 is 2 mg. Good dietary sources include whole-grains, liver, meat, egg yolk, oily fish, soy and dark green, leafy vegetables.

Vitamin B12

Lack of vitamin B12 lessens the activity of bone building cells (osteoblasts) and may lead to reduced bone strength and osteoporosis. The EU RDA for vitamin B12 is 1 mcg. Vitamin B12 is mainly found in animal-based foods, such as liver, kidney, fish, red meat, eggs and dairy products. Preparations of vitamin B12 made by bacterial fermentation – and therefore acceptable to vegetarians – are available.

Folic Acid

Folic acid helps to prevent a build up of an amino acid, homocysteine, that promotes both osteoporosis and coronary heart disease. Around one in ten people inherit higher than normal blood levels of homocysteine, which triples the risk of these diseases. One in 160,000 people have extremely high levels, with 30 times the risk of premature heart disease and osteoporosis. See page 72 for further information.

Essential Fatty Acids

A diet rich in certain essential fatty acids (EFAs) seems to stimulate calcium uptake from the gut, decrease calcium loss in the urine and trigger increased calcium deposition in bone. Increasing your intake of essential fatty acids, as well as boosting your calcium intake, will help to protect against osteoporosis. For more information, see pages 153–6.

Saturated Fats

A high intake of saturated fat reduces absorption of two important bone minerals from the gut – calcium and magnesium. As a result, a high fat diet is linked with loss of calcium from the body and an increased risk of osteoporotic fractures. For more information, see page 104.

Salt

A diet that contains excessive salt increases the risk of osteoporosis as well as high blood pressure. Excess sodium increases the loss of calcium in urine. You can therefore reduce your risk of osteoporosis by cutting down your salt intake. Research suggests that halving the average salt intake could cut calcium loss in the urine by as much as 20 per cent. Ideally, you should obtain no more than 4–6 g salt (sodium chloride) per day from your diet. See pages 118–9 for more details.

Sugar

A high sugar intake increases the loss of the minerals calcium, chromium, copper, magnesium and zinc from the body. It is therefore important to limit dietary sugars when taking steps to help prevent osteoporosis.

Caffeine

Caffeine increases the loss of calcium and magnesium in the urine, increases production of parathyroid hormone and lowers blood calcium levels which together increase the amount of calcium absorbed from bone. Just 300 mg caffeine

– found in two large cups of filter coffee – can cause the loss of an extra 15 mg calcium from the body. This could contribute to as much as a 10 per cent fall in bone mass over a ten-year period after the menopause. As a result, women who drink four cups of coffee per day are three times more likely to suffer a hip fracture at some stage in their life. Some experts suggest that women should obtain an extra 40 g calcium for every 6 fl oz (178 ml) serving of caffeine-containing coffee consumed. Try switching to decaffeinated brands of tea and coffee, avoid caffeinated fizzy drink such as cola and boost your calcium intake to compensate for the amount of caffeine you do consume.

Reducing Menopausal Symptoms through Diet

Nutrition plays a major role in helping to reduce menopausal symptoms such as hot flushes, night sweats and fatigue. The old saying 'We are what we eat' applies at all times of life, but perhaps even more so now, as hormone balance can be affected by:

- the types of fat you eat
- how much fibre you eat
- the amount of natural plant hormones (phytoestrogens) present in your food
- the amount of vitamins, minerals and trace elements you obtain

The Effects of a High-fat, Low-fibre Diet

Women who have followed the typical unhealthy Western diet that is high in fat and meat and low in fibre have relatively high levels of circulating oestrogen before the menopause, which is believed to increase the risk of certain hormone-dependent tumours such as breast cancer. Once the menopause is reached, however, and these high oestrogen levels fall, more severe menopausal symptoms can occur – the tissues have become used to a relatively high level of circulating hormones, and seem to tolerate the menopausal drop less well. It is also more difficult for the body's normal coping mechanisms (e.g. the adrenal glands, see page 219) to compensate for the comparatively large difference between pre- and post-menopausal oestrogen exposure.

Switching to a healthier, low-fat, high-fibre diet around the time of the menopause can also make symptoms of oestrogen withdrawal worse by lowering natural oestrogen levels even further. This is because dietary fibre absorbs oestrogen hormones present in the bile so that rather than being reabsorbed into the body, they are excreted along with the fibre instead. Unless you have problems with constipation, it is a good idea not to suddenly increase your intake of fibre at this time of life, but to increase it little by little, and also to compensate by eating a diet rich in oestrogen-like plant hormones known as phytoestrogens.

Fibre

Dietary fibre is made up of the indigestible parts of plants foods that we cannot break down and absorb during digestion. It therefore stays in the intestinal tract to help encourage the muscular, wave-like bowel movements that push digested food through your system.

Average intakes of fibre are low, at around 20 g per day, and most women would benefit from slowly increasing their intake of fibre from a variety of fruit and vegetable sources, to the recommended level of around 30 g per day. Although fibre from natural sources is beneficial, taking too much fibre – usually as a result of taking fibre supplements – can make menopausal symptoms worse. This is because it binds oestrogen hormones secreted into the bile from the liver, so they are excreted rather than being re-absorbed back into the circulation. Unless you have problems with constipation, it is therefore not a good idea to take fibre supplements on a long-term basis, but to increase the amount of fruit and vegetables (which are also rich in plant hormones) instead.

The main sources of dietary fibre are unrefined complex carbohydrates such as wholemeal bread, wholegrain cereals, wholewheat pasta, brown rice, nuts, seeds, pulses, vegetables and fresh or dried fruits.

Bran-containing breakfast cereals provide one of the highest concentrations of dietary fibre.

Good Dietary Sources of Fibre:

- Bran provides 40 g fibre per 100 g portion
- Dried apricots 18 g per 100 g
- Peas 5 g per 100 g
- Prunes 13 g per 100 g
- Cooked brown rice 4 g per 100 g
- Cooked wholemeal spaghetti 4 g per 100 g
- Brown bread 6 g per 100 g
- Walnuts 6 g per 100 g

Phytoestrogens

Many plants contain natural chemicals that have a weak, hormone-like action in the human body. These plant hormones, known as phytoestrogens, can help to compensate for falling hormone levels after the menopause, reduce short- and medium-term menopausal symptoms. Perhaps more importantly, they also help to protect against long-term problems associated with oestrogen-withdrawal such as osteoporosis and coronary heart disease (see pages 94 and 78 for further information).

Because they help to normalize the body's oestrogen levels, which the menopause depletes, phytoestrogens are often referred to as natural hormone replacement therapy.

Phytoestrogens are plant hormones that have a similar structure to human oestrogens, but are 500 to 1,000 times less active as oestrogen receptors. They are present in the diet in three main forms:

- isoflavones (e.g. genistein, daidzein, formononetin, biochanin A and glycitein) are found in members of the pea and bean family such as soy and chickpeas
- flavonoids are present in high concentrations in many fruits and vegetables, especially apples and onions – and also found in green and black tea leaves
- lignans are found mainly in linseed but also in sesame seeds, wholegrain cereals, fruit and vegetables.

Phytoestrogens have a number of important, beneficial physiological effects in the human body. They can damp down high oestrogen states by competing for the stronger natural oestrogens to occupy landing sites on oestrogen receptors within body cells. This reduces the amount of oestrogen stimulation a cell receives (it gets stimulation from a weak plant oestrogen in place of a strong human oestrogen) and is thought to help protect against breast cancer (see page 152). As they have a weak oestrogen action, phytoestrogens also provide an additional hormone boost when oestrogen levels are low after the menopause. They are therefore often referred to as natural hormone replacement therapy.

ISOFLAVONES

Isoflavones are the most extensively studied phytoestrogens. Isoflavones are a group of non-steroidal plant hormones (phytoestrogens) that have a similar structure to human oestradiol. Plant isoflavones are mostly present in the in-active (glycosylated) form in which they are bound to a sugar molecule. After being eaten, however, intestinal bacteria break them down by removing the sugar residue, which converts them into their activated forms. These are then absorbed into the circulation and taken straight to the liver.

Around a thousand different plant isoflavones have been identified, but only five with oestrogenic activity are normally obtained from our diet in significant amounts. These are: genistein, daidzein and glycitein (obtained mainly from soy products) plus formononetin and biochanin A (which are metabolized to form daidzein and genistein in the body), obtained mostly from chickpeas, lentils and mung beans.

The traditional Japanese diet is low in fat, especially satu-rated fat, and consists of rice, soy products (e.g. soybeans, soymeal, tofu) and fish together with legumes, grains and yellow-green vegetables such as cruciferous plants. These include exotic members of the cabbage and turnip families (e.g. kohlrabi, Chinese leaves). Soy and cruciferous plants are a rich source of isoflavones and in Japan where soya is a dietary staple, intakes of isoflavones are 50 to 100 mg per day – 20 to 30 times higher than typical western intakes of just 2–5 mg isoflavones per day. Blood levels of phytoestrogen are therefore as much as 110 times higher in Japanese women of menopausal age than those typically found in the West. As a result, less than a quarter of Japanese women complain of hot flushes in middle age, compared with four out of five women in the US. This is not a genetic effect, for when Japanese people move to the West and follow a typical Western diet, their blood hormone levels and risk of illnesses such as coronary heart disease and breast cancer eventually become similar to those of the local population, and their susceptibility to menopausal symptoms also increases.

PHYTOESTROGENS AND CORONARY HEART DISEASE

Phytoestrogens have a beneficial effect on the circulation by helping to maintain elasticity of arterial walls, to dilate coronary arteries, increase the pumping action of the heart and reduce harmful LDL cholesterol levels. The way they lower harmful LDL cholesterol levels is unknown, but some researchers think they increase the activity of LDL receptors on cells, so more is taken up into cells and burned as fuel, or that less LDL cholesterol is made in the liver. In addition, phytoestrogens lower blood stickiness, have beneficial anti-oxidant and anti-inflammatory activity and may possibly raise beneficial HDL cholesterol levels. Studies have also suggested that phytoestrogens can inhibit overgrowth of cells found in the walls and lining of arteries, and reduce unwanted blood clot formation. Taken together, these actions may help to explain why the Japanese, with their high level of dietary phytoestrogens, have one of the lowest rates of coronary heart disease in the world. Based on scientific evidence from over 50 independent studies, the US Food and Drug Administration (FDA) have allowed manufacturers to make health claims on food labels that 'A diet low in saturated fat and cholesterol, and which includes 25 g soya protein per day, can significantly reduce the risk of coronary heart disease.'

PHYTOESTROGENS AND OSTEOPOROSIS

Like conventional hormone replacement therapy, phyto-estrogens have been shown to have a beneficial effect on bones, increasing the activity of bone-building cells (osteoblasts) and reducing the activity of bone-dissolving cells (osteoclasts) so that more new bone is produced, and less old bone is broken down. A daily intake of 2.25 mg isoflavones from isolated soya protein has been shown to significantly increase bone mineral content and density in the lumbar spine and to protect against osteoporosis of the spine. In fact, a study involving 650 women aged 19 to 86 found those with the highest intake of dietary phytoestro-gens (assessed using a food frequency questionnaire) had significantly stronger bones after the menopause (bone mineral density 0.820 versus 0.771 g/cm) after adjusting for age, height, weight, years since menopause, smoking, alcohol consumption, HRT usage and daily calcium intake. The researchers suggested that a high isoflavone intake may help to reduce the rate at which bone thins after the menopause by reversing over-activity of hyperparathyroid glands (which raise blood calcium levels by leaching it out of bones) which is associated with oestrogen withdrawal in postmenopausal women. Phytoestrogens therefore offer a real alternative to HRT for women who are unable or unwilling to take it.

PHYTOESTROGENS AND BREAST CANCER

Prescribed HRT usually has to be limited so that a woman takes it for a maximum of ten years (counting from the age of 50) to help minimize any possible increased risk of breast cancer. In contrast, research suggests that phytoestrogens may play an important role in protecting against breast cancer. Isoflavones can reduce the activity of tumour growth factors (so tumours receive less growth stimulation), reduce the formation of new blood vessels within tumours (so they are starved of oxygen and nutrients). They are also believed to protect genetic material from some of the damage that may trigger cancer in the first place. A study of 406 women aged 45–74 years found that those with the highest soy intake were least likely to have the breast changes seen on mammography that are associated with a high risk of future breast cancer. Those eating most soy were 60 per cent less likely to have a high risk of breast cancer than those eating the least. It has also been suggested that increased isoflavone intake reduces the risk of breast cancer in younger women through beneficial effects on oestrogen metabolism, hormone concentrations and menstrual cycle length

Phytoestrogens are a beneficial dietary component, and high dietary intakes among men, women and children appear to have no obvious adverse effects (but see warnings regarding isoflavone supplements, page 184).

DIETARY SOURCES OF PHYTOESTROGENS
As phytoestrogens have such a wide range of beneficial effects, it is important to consider increasing your intake at all stages of life, but especially after the menopause. Aim to increase your intake of fruit and vegetables, which contain plant hormones.

Sources of phytoestrogens

- Legumes: soy beans and soy products such as tofu, tempeh, miso, tamari, lentils .
- Vegetables: dark green leafy vegetables (e.g. broccoli, Pak choi, spinach) and exotic members of the cruciferous family (e.g. Chinese leaves, kohlrabi); celery, fennel
- Fresh fruits: apples, avocados, bananas, mangoes, papayas, rhubarb
- Dried fruits: dates, figs, prunes, raisins
- Wholegrains: almost all, especially corn, buckwheat, millet, oats, rye, wheat
- Nuts: almonds, cashew nuts, hazelnuts, peanuts, walnuts and nut oils
- Seeds: almost all, especially linseeds, pumpkin seeds, sesame seeds, sunflower seeds and sprouted seeds (e.g. alfalfa, mung beans, lentils, red clover, soya beans)
- Culinary herbs: especially angelica, chervil, chives, garlic, ginger, horseradish, nutmeg, parsley, rosemary, sage, seaweed (kelp, Irish moss), nettles and watercress
- Honey: especially that made from wild flowers.

One of the main dietary sources of isoflavones is soya, which is rich in daidzein, genistein and glycitein. Sixty gm of soy protein provides as much as 45 mg isoflavones. Soya is an acquired taste, however, and is not always easy to incorporate into the Western diet, despite the increased availability of functional foods enriched with phytoestrogens, such as breads and muesli bars. Supplements providing isoflavones extracted from non-GMO soya beans, Japanese Arrowroot (Kudzu) or Red Clover are therefore becoming increasingly popular (see Chapter 9).

Essential Fatty Acids

Essential fatty acids (EFAs) are so called because they cannot be made in large quantities in the body and it is therefore essential that they should be supplied by your diet. There are two main EFAs:

- linoleic acid (an omega-6 polyunsaturated fatty acid)
- linolenic acid (an omega-3 polyunsaturated fatty acid)

Both linoleic and linolenic acids are found in rich quantities in walnuts, pumpkin seeds, soybeans, linseed (flaxseed) oil and rapeseed oil. Linoleic acid alone is found in sunflower seed, almonds, corn, sesame seed, safflower oil and extra virgin olive oil, while linolenic acid alone is found in evening primrose oil, starflower (borage) seed oil and blackcurrant seed oils (available as food supplements – see Chapter 9).

Once in your body, these EFAs act as building blocks to make sex hormones, including oestrogen, as well as hormone-like chemicals known as prostaglandins. They are also important for healthy cell membranes throughout the body, especially those found in the skin and nervous system. A diet that supplies optimal levels of essential fatty acids is vital at all times of life, but especially around the time of the menopause and beyond.

Unfortunately, a dietary lack of EFAs is common, and the way your metabolism handles those available can also be blocked by a variety of diet and lifestyle factors that can contribute to deficiency, including:

- eating too much saturated fat which is mainly supplied from animal sources
- eating too many trans-fatty acids (found in some hydrogenated margarines)
- eating too much sugar
- drinking too much alcohol

- deficiency of vitamins and minerals, especially vitamin B6, zinc and magnesium
- crash dieting
- smoking cigarettes
- exposure to pollution
- excessive stress.

If your diet is lacking in EFAs, your metabolism can make do with the next best fatty acids available, such as those derived from saturated fats, but this is not ideal as it leads to the production of cell membranes that are more rigid and more prone to dryness, itching and premature ageing than when EFAs were in plentiful supply.

Cell membranes also contain receptors that interact with circulating hormones such as oestrogen, and if you lack EFAs at this time of life, your hormones may not be able to interact with tissues – including those in the bones and circulation – as well as they should.

EFAs also act as building blocks for sex hormones, and dietary deficiency can lead to hormone and prostaglandin imbalances that may contribute to menopausal symptoms, dry itchy skin, irregular periods and osteoporosis. The EFAs that appear to be most beneficial at this time of life are gammalinolenic acid (GLA – found in evening primrose, starflower, flaxseed and hemp seed oils) and eicosapentaenoic acid (EPA – found mainly in oily fish).

To boost your intake of EFAs, aim to eat more:

- Nuts and seeds – sprinkle onto cereals, yoghurt, desserts and salads
- Bread enriched with soybeans and linseed (flaxseed)
- Dark green, leafy vegetables
- Oily fish such as mackerel, herring, salmon, trout, sardines and pilchards (tuna is not classed as oily, but still contains beneficial oils) – aim for at least 300 g per week, preferably from organic sources to avoid excess levels of pollutants
- Sunflower, olive and rapessed oils in cooking and salad dressings
- Evening Primrose Oil as a supplement (see pages 173–4)

An Organic Diet

Organic fruit, vegetables, dairy products and livestock are grown or reared using farming practices that involve minimal use of chemicals, and have been subjected to minimal processing. Organic practices are proven and sustainable methods of producing food in harmony with nature, without the use of pesticides, weed killers, fungicides, fumigants, growth promoters, growth retardants, antibiotics, hormones, artificial fertilizers, genetic manipulation, irradiation or undue exposure to environmental pollution. In their place, farmers use traditional methods of pest control, crop rotation, growing green manure crops (e.g. clover), careful timing of sowing and allowing land to lie fallow.

One of the main benefits of organic foods is that they contain minimal levels of agricultural chemicals, whose effects on health are not fully understood. Some of these chemicals are known to have certain hormone-like actions in the body, and are believed to have affected the gender and reproductive functions of some forms of wildlife.

Whether or not non-organic foods can affect the timing

of the menopause, or worsen menopausal symptoms, is currently unknown, but many women choose to follow an organic diet. This does seem to have a beneficial effect on their general well-being at this time of life.

Another benefit of organic foods is that they tend to contain significantly more vitamins, minerals, trace elements, EFAs, fibre and other important protective substances such as phytoestrogens than commercially grown produce. This is partly because they contain less water and more solid matter, but also due to the quality of the replenished soils in which they are grown. Non-organic crops are frequently grown in artificially fertilized soils boosted with nitrogen, phosphorus and potassium, but depleted of other minerals and trace elements such as selenium, which are not replenished. Spraying with pesticides and other chemicals may interfere with the nutrient content of plants, especially when present in certain combinations, while fruit and vegetables shipped from abroad are often picked before ripe so their nutrient content is naturally low.

In the UK, organic standards are set by an EC directive. Organic foods are checked and certified by an independent body such as the Soil Association (see Useful Addresses) to ensure producers stick to a strict code of practice.

Liquids

Fluid is just as essential for good health as what you eat. Aim to drink at least 3 litres of fluid per day. Mineral water is a good source of calcium for your bones, too, especially in hard water areas.

Glycaemic index

Dietary carbohydrates are made up of simple sugars (e.g. glucose) and complex carbohydrates. Simple sugars quickly raise blood sugar levels, to give a short-term energy boost. Complex carbohydrates (e.g. starch) are made up of chains of simple sugars, and must first be broken down into these units before they can act as an energy source.

The way in which different foods make your blood glucose levels rise is known as their glycaemic index (GI). For optimum energy levels and general health, it is best to eat foods with a low to moderate GI, and to combine foods with a high GI (e.g. potatoes) with those that have a lower GI (e.g. beans) to help even out fluctuations in blood glucose levels.

The following chart shows the glycaemic index of a variety of foods compared with glucose, which has the highest glycaemic index of 100.

High Glycaemic Foods	GI
Glucose	100
Baked potatoes	98
Parsnips	97
White bread	95
Carrots	92
Popcorn	85
Brown rice	82
Cornflakes	80
Weetabix	75
Wholemeal bread	72
Boiled potatoes	70
Chocolate bar	68
Shredded wheat	67

Raisins	64
Bananas	62
Cheese pizza	60
Chocolate biscuit	59
Rich Tea biscuit	57
Basmati rice	58
Porridge oats	54
Crisps	51
Cake	50

Low Glycaemic Foods	GI
Baked beans	48
Peas	48
Grapes	44
Muesli	43
Wholemeal pasta	42
All Bran	42
Oranges	40
Apples	39
Fish fingers	38
Ice cream	36
Low fat yoghurt	33
Milk	32
Strawberries	32
Apricots	31
Beans and lentils	30
Sausages	28
Grapefruit	25
Cherries	24
Soya beans	18
Green leafy vegetables	15
Mushrooms	9

Interestingly, the food contributing most to a high glycemic load in one study was baked potatoes – traditionally thought of as the dieter's friend! To switch to a low GI diet, consider eating:

- breakfast cereals based on wheat bran, barley and oats
- grainy breads made with whole seeds
- pasta and rice in place of potatoes.

Putting it all Together: a Healthy Diet for the Menopause

A healthy diet can help to reduce the severity of menopausal symptoms as well as helping to reduce the risk of age-related conditions that become more prevalent in later life (see Chapter 6). If you follow the dietary tips outlined in this chapter, you will undoubtedly be eating more healthily and combating many symptoms and conditions associated with the menopause.

Sample Diet Plan

Here is a simple, one-week eating plan to give you an idea how you can adapt the principles suggested in this chapter into a healthy menopausal diet.

DAY 1

BREAKFAST   Slice melon

Unsweetened muesli with 4 chopped dried apricots and semi-skimmed milk

Fresh, unsweetened orange juice

Mid-Morning   Small banana

LUNCH   Green tagliatelle
                     Grilled salmon with lemon, garlic and dill
                     Steamed spinach
                     Steamed broccoli

                     Stewed, unsweetened rhubarb with low-fat vanilla
                     fromage frais

Mid-Afternoon   Apple

DINNER   Ciabatta, focaccia or fresh bread with soya and
                     linseed
                     Hummus
                     1 large beef tomato
                     Mixed salad: Chinese leaves, celery, fennel and
                     walnuts sprinkled with a tablespoon of mixed seeds
                     (sunflower, pumpkin, sesame, poppy)

                     Low-fat Bio yoghurt with chopped fresh peach and a
                     few almonds

Evening   Glass of red wine or red grape juice
                     Handful of grapes
                     Herbal tea (e.g. fennel)

DAY 2

BREAKFAST   Slice melon
                     1 slice brown bread or fresh bread with soya and
                     linseed
                     Scraping butter/low fat spread and reduced sugar
                     marmalade
                     Unsweetened grapefruit juice

Mid-Morning   Nectarine

LUNCH   Small baked potato

Aubergine parmesan

Mixed green salad leaves, green and yellow peppers, fennel and grated carrot

Large orange

Mid-Afternoon   Apple

DINNER   Granary roll or fresh bread with soya and linseed
Fennel and bean salad
Large mixed salad with 60 g Feta cheese and a few hazelnuts

Low-fat fromage frais with chopped banana and a few walnuts

Evening   Glass of red wine or red grape juice
Handful of grapes
Herbal tea: (e.g. Raspberry and ginseng)

DAY 3

BREAKFAST   4 large prunes soaked overnight in Lapsang Souchong tea
Low-fat Bio yoghurt (vanilla)
1 slice brown toast or fresh bread with soya and linseed
Scraping butter/low-fat spread and marmalade
Fresh, unsweetened orange juice

Mid-Morning   Peach

LUNCH   Granary bread, ciabatta, focaccia or fresh bread with soya and linseed
Roasted stuffed red peppers
Steamed green beans
Steamed baby carrots and baby sweet corn

Fresh kiwi fruit with low-fat fromage frais

Mid-Afternoon   Small banana

DINNER   2 slices pumpernickel or fresh bread with soya and linseed
Low-fat cottage cheese with a slice of fresh pineapple
½ avocado
Mixed salad with Chinese leaves, flat leaved parsley, coriander leaves, fennel, grated carrot and green/yellow peppers

Low-fat fromage frais with chopped walnuts and Acacia honey

Evening   Glass of red wine or red grape juice
Handful of grapes
Herbal tea: (e.g. apple and blackberry)

DAY 4
BREAKFAST   ½ grilled pink grapefruit
Unsweetened muesli with 4 dried apricots and semi-skimmed milk
Unsweetened grapefruit juice

Mid-Morning   Small banana

LUNCH   Brown rice
Chicken with Lemon and Olives
Steamed spinach
Steamed mangetout

Stewed or fresh plums with fromage frais

Mid-Afternoon   Apple

DINNER   Pitta or fresh bread with soya and linseed
Pesto rice salad

Green lentil, ginger and coriander salad

Mixed green salad leaves and ½ avocado

Low-fat fromage frais with chopped nectarine and mixed nuts

Evening
Glass of red wine or red grape juice

Handful of grapes

Herbal tea (e.g. camomile and lemon grass)

DAY 5

BREAKFAST
Half pink grapefruit

1 slice brown toast or fresh bread with soya and linseed

Scraping of butter/low-fat spread with yeast extract

Unsweetened orange juice

Mid-Morning
Pear

LUNCH
Ciabatta, focaccia or fresh bread with soya and linseed

Pasta with chargrilled Mediterranean Vegetables

Mixed green salad with a tblsp mixed seeds

Low-fat Bio yoghurt with chopped walnuts and Acacia honey

Mid-Afternoon
Apple

DINNER
Granary roll or fresh bread with soya and linseed

Home-made mushroom, garlic and fennel soup

Walnut and coriander pâté

Handful of watercress

2 Rye crispbreads

Bowl of cherries with low-fat fromage frais

Evening
Glass of red wine or red grape juice

Handful of grapes

Herbal tea (e.g. lemon verbena)

DAY 6

BREAKFAST   Slice melon

1 slice brown toast or fresh bread with soya and linseed

Mushrooms fried with garlic and a little low-fat olive-oil based spread

Fresh cranberry juice

Mid-Morning   Apple

LUNCH   Ciabatta, foccacia or fresh bread with soya and linseed

Grilled trout with almonds

Grilled beef tomatoes, steamed broccoli

Steamed green beans

Low-fat fromage frais with raspberries

Mid-Afternoon   Small banana

DINNER   Ciabatta, Foccacia or fresh bread with soya and linseed

Mediterranean Bean Soup

Orange and pink grapefruit slices

Evening   Glass of red wine or red grape juice

Handful of grapes

Herbal tea (e.g. ginger)

DAY 7

BREAKFAST   Slice melon

2 slices brown toast or fresh bread with soya and linseed

Butter or low-fat olive-oil based spread

Smoked salmon with freshly squeezed lemon juice

Fresh cranberry juice

Mid-Morning   Orange

LUNCH   Roast Lamb with rosemary, garlic and cannellini beans
Roast red pepper and Florence fennel (brush with
olive oil for roasting)
Roast potatoes and parsnips (brush with olive oil for
roasting)
Spring greens

Home-made mint-sauce (fresh mint, Balsamic vinegar,
pinch brown sugar)

Gooseberry fool made with low-fat fromage frais

Mid-Afternoon   Apple

DINNER   Granary roll, ciabatta or fresh bread with soya and
linseed
Tomato, orange and ginger soup

Low fat Bio yoghurt with melon balls

Evening   Glass of red wine or red grape juice
Handful of grapes
Herbal tea (e.g. marigold)

9
Nutritional Supplements and their Benefits

Several vitamins, minerals, essential fatty acid and herbal supplements are widely taken by women as the menopause approaches as seen in the previous chapter on diet. Some act as a nutritional safety net to help maintain general health and well-being, while others have a beneficial effect on menopausal symptoms such as hot flushes, night sweats and emotional changes.

Multivitamins and Minerals

Surveys suggest that many women do not obtain all the vitamins and minerals they need from their diet. Even if only one nutrient is in short supply, it can affect your metabolism, immune system and hormonal balance and have the potential to worsen menopausal symptoms.

While diet should always come first, a good multivitamin and mineral supplement acts as a nutritional safety net. Choose a supplement according to your age, as after the menopausal age of 50 to 55, your need for many vitamins and minerals increases. This is partly because your metabolism needs more, and partly because changes in the intestinal wall mean you are less able to absorb certain nutrients from your diet. Look at the labels to see how each supplement compares. If you are under 50, select one providing at least 100 per cent of the recommended daily amount (RDA) of as many vitamins and minerals as possible. Those designed for people over the age of 50 will generally contain more antioxidants and B group vitamins, but less iron, as body stores of this mineral increase in later life and excess may be harmful.

For information on antioxidants and their protective effect against coronary heart disease and information on vitamins and minerals that help to prevent osteoporosis, see Chapter 8.

Agnus Castus (Vitex agnus castus)

Agnus castus fruits contain substances that have a progesterone-like action in women. It has been shown to decrease secretion of follicle stimulating hormone (FSH), which makes it helpful for treating menopausal symptoms – especially hot flushes and night sweats – which are indirectly linked with increased levels of FSH.

Some women experience worsening symptoms of premenstrual syndrome (PMS) as the menopause approaches, and in a recent study of 170 women with PMS, there was a greater than 50 per cent improvement in overall symptoms in those taking Agnus castus, compared with this level of improvement in only 24 per cent of those taking placebo. It is especially helpful for symptoms of headache, breast tenderness, bloating, fatigue and emotional symptoms such as restlessness, anxiety, depression, irritability, anger, mood swings and lack of concentration.

Dose: Tablets – 500 mg daily (extracts standardized to contain 0.5 per cent agnuside: 175 to 225 mg daily). It is usually taken as a single daily dose first thing in the morning. It is slow acting and may take a month to show effects. The average length of treatment is six months.

Note: Vitex agnus castus should not be taken during pregnancy, or at the same time as other hormone treatments such as HRT and hormonal methods of contraception. Excess can cause a crawling sensation on the skin.

Black Cohosh (Cimicifuga racemosa)

Black Cohosh is valued for its hormone and mood balancing properties. Its dried root contains a number of oestrogen-like plant hormones (phytoestrogens) of which formononetin is thought to be the most important. It also has a direct action on centres of the brain that help to control dilation of blood vessels, which helps to reduce menopausal hot flushes and sweating.

Black Cohosh is one of the most widely used and studied natural alternatives to hormone replacement therapy (HRT). Standardized extracts have been shown to produce beter results in relieving hot flushes, vaginal thinning and dryness, depression and anxiety compared to standard HRT (conjugated oestrogens). In one study, Black Cohosh out-performed diazepam and oestrogen HRT in relieving depressive moods and anxiety.

It is sometimes combined with St John's Wort and one trial found that the two herbs together were effective in reducing hot flushes and other menopausal symptoms in 78 per cent of women taking it – improvements usually start to occur within two to four weeks. No serious side-effects have been reported. Some people have experienced headaches behind the eyes, nausea, or indigestion if they have taken too much Black Cohosh.

As Black Cohosh has a normalizing effect on female sex hormones, it is also useful for improving low sex drive, which can sometimes occur at this time of life (see Chapter 14).

Dose: usually 80 mg to 160 mg standardized extracts daily.

Note: Black Cohosh should not be taken during pregnancy or when breast-feeding. It has been used in women with a history of breast cancer, although this should only be done under the supervision of a qualified herbalist.

Cranberry (Vaccinium macrocarpon)

Cranberries contain substances known as anti-adhesins, which help to stop bacteria (especially Escherichia coli, the commonest cause of urinary tract infections) from sticking to cells lining the urinary tract wall. As a result, they are more easily flushed out, and taking cranberry extracts or drinking cranberry juice helps to reduce the incidence of urinary symptoms after the menopause.

Drinking just half a pint of cranberry juice daily can almost halve the risk of developing cystitis. In a ground-breaking clinical trial involving over 150 older women, those drinking 300 ml cranberry juice per day for six months were 42 per cent less likely to develop pus cells in their urine than those drinking a synthetic placebo that was indistinguishable in taste, appearance and vitamin C content but which lacked cranberry extracts. Furthermore, if pus cells did develop in the urine, the chance of infection still being present after one month was only 27 per cent of the odds in those not drinking cranberry juice.

Cranberry fruit solids also have beneficial anti-adhesin properties and in a clinical trial involving 24 women with recurrent urinary tract infections, those taking cranberry supplements for six months had significantly fewer urinary tract infections than those taking prophylactic antibiotics.

Cranberry is also helpful for reducing the unpleasant odours associated with urinary incontinence.

Dose: Cranberry juice 300 ml daily. Cranberry supplements: 500 mg daily.

Note: If you think you may have a urinary infection, seek medical advice if symptoms do not improve within a day or two.

Dandelion (Taraxacum officinalis)

Dandelion is one of the most widely used herbal remedies. It stimulates removal of toxins from the body and is a powerful diuretic as well as being a rich source of the mineral potassium. It helps to flush excess sodium salts and fluid through the kidneys. It is a useful treatment for the fluid retention that can occur with pre-menstrual bloating around the time of the menopause and may also help to reduce the unpleasant effects of night sweats. Interestingly, dandelion does not seem to have a diuretic action in those with a normal healthy fluid balance who do not need to lose excess water.

As it promotes absorption of dietary iron, it is sometimes used to treat anaemia.

Dose: 500 mg extracts twice a day.

Note: Side-effects are uncommon, but large doses can cause nausea and diarrhoea. Do not use if you have active gall-stones or obstructive jaundice.

Dong Quai (Angelica sinensis)

Dong Quai (Chinese angelica) is a popular female tonic. Its rhizome contains oestrogen-like phytoestrogens that help to provide a useful additional oestrogen boost when levels start to fall at the menopause. Unfortunately, a 12-week clinical study involving 71 women did not find a significant improvement in menopausal symptoms among those taking Dong Quai on its own, and those taking inactive placebo. This does not prove lack of efficacy, however, as Chinese angelica is usually prescribed in combination with other herbs such as Agnus castus, liquorice and Siberian ginseng, with which it may have a synergistic action.

Dong Quai does seem to be effective in easing menstrual cramps, which can prove troublesome as the menopause approaches (see page 13). In one study, Dong Quai was 1.7 times more effective as an analgesic than aspirin for relieving painful muscle spasms. It is also used to improve headaches, to support ovarian function and to regulate an irregular menstrual cycle.

Dose: Capsules standardized to 9000 ppm ligustilide: 200 mg three times daily.

Note: No serious side-effects have been reported at standard doses. It may cause a skin rash on exposure to sun in some people, especially those with fair skin. Angelica has an anti-blood clotting action and should be avoided by women who experience heavy menstruation, abnormal bleeding or who take anticoagulants such as warfarin or aspirin regularly. Do not take if you have peptic ulcers, during pregnancy or breast-feeding.

Evening Primrose Oil

The seeds of the Evening Primrose are a rich source of gammalinolenic acid (GLA). GLA is metabolized in the body to form hormone-like substances known as prostaglandins. These help to maintain a healthy hormone balance, and Evening Primrose Oil (EPO) can help a wide range of problems including dry itchy skin, premenstrual syndrome and menopausal symptoms.

The action of GLA is boosted by vitamin E, which also helps to preserve it. Certain vitamins and minerals are also needed during the metabolism of essential fatty acids. These are vitamin C, vitamin B6, vitamin B3 (niacin), zinc and magnesium. If you are taking Evening Primrose Oil, you should therefore ensure that your intake of these is adequate.

Dose: 1000 mg EPO daily for general health (equivalent to 80 mg GLA). Up to 3 g daily (equivalent to 240 mg GLA) may be taken to treat hormone imbalances (e.g. associated with cyclical breast pain, pre-menstrual syndrome or menopausal symptoms). It can take up to 3 months to notice a beneficial effect, however. As an oil, it is best taken with food to boost absorption. 1000 mg starflower (borage) oil is equivalent to 3000 mg evening primrose oil or 1500 mg blackcurrant seed oil.

Note: The only people who should not take EPO are those who are allergic to it and those with a particular nervous disorder known as temporal lobe epilepsy.

False Unicorn (Chamaelirium luteum; Helonias dioica)

False Unicorn is perennial herb, native to North America, which is also known as Blazing Star and Fairy Wand. Its root is a powerful stimulant and normalizer of the female reproductive system, as it contains up to 9 per cent oestrogen-like steroidal saponins similar to those found in ginseng, plus glycosides such as chamaelirin and helonin. Little research has been performed on this interesting herb, but it is used to treat gynaecological problems as it has a balancing effect on oestrogen. It contains chemicals that compete with oestrogen receptors to help damp down the effects of excess oestrogen production, but also provides additional oestrogen activity where natural oestrogen levels are low. It encourages a normal menstrual cycle and has been used to help prevent and treat menopausal symptoms. It is especially useful for women who have a tendency toward pelvic congestion with sensations of heaviness, tiredness, backache and low mood associated with the menopause. It is said to be especially helpful for early symptoms of the menopause

Dose: Tincture: 10 drops, 3 times a day. It can take several months for False Unicorn to have an effect, so it is usually taken for long courses.

Note: High doses can cause nausea and vomiting.

Garlic (Allium sativum)

Garlic has a number of medicinal uses but its most important effect is its ability to maintain a healthy circulation and reduce the risk of coronary heart disease and stroke – conditions that become more common in women after the menopause. The main substance derived from garlic that protects against CHD is allicin, which gives a crushed clove its characteristic smell.

Taking standardized garlic extracts can reduce high blood pressure, lower levels of harmful blood fats (LDL cholesterol and triglycerides – see Chapter 8), reduce blood stickiness and clotting to improve circulation. Garlic has a beneficial effect on the circulation due to a number of different actions. It can:

- prevent cells from taking up cholesterol and reduce cholesterol production in the liver
- decrease blood stickiness and clot formation
- dissolve unwanted blood clots
- dilate blood vessels by relaxing smooth muscle cells
- increase the elasticity of the aorta so the heart has to work less hard to pump blood out into the body.

Enteric coating of garlic powder tablets reduces garlic odour on breath and protects the active ingredients from degradation in the stomach.

Dose: 600 to 900 mg daily.

Ginseng (Panax ginseng)

Ginseng roots contain unique substances known as ginseno-sides, of which 29 have been identified. Some, classed as Rb1 ginsenosides, have a calming action, while others – known as Rg1 ginsenosides – are more stimulating.

Many of the steroidal compounds it contains are similar in structure to human sex hormones and Ginseng has a normalizing effect on hormone imbalances. Ginseng also helps to stimulate the adrenal glands to increase their output of corticosteroids and sex hormones (usually around 5 per cent of circulating sex hormones such as testosterone are produced by the adrenal glands). It is stimulating and restorative, improving physical and mental energy levels, and helps the body adapt to physical or emotional stress and fatigue. Ginseng is also prized as an aphrodisiac. It is one of the most effective adaptogens – herbs that help the body adapt to physical and emotional stress – for women approaching the menopause and beyond.

Dose: Depends on grade of root. Choose a standardized product, preferably with a content of at least 5 per cent ginsenosides. Start with a low dose and work up from 200–1000 mg per day. The optimum dose is usually around 600 mg daily. In the East, ginseng is taken in a two-weeks on, two-weeks off cycle. Some practitioners recommend taking it in a 6 weeks-on, 8 weeks-off cycle.

Note: Ginseng is not advised if you have high blood pressure (as it may make hypertension worse), a heart rhythm abnor-mality or if you have an oestrogen dependent condition (e.g. pregnancy, cancer of the breast, ovaries or uterus). Hormonal effects, such as postmenopausal bleeding and painful breasts (mastalgia) in older women, have also been reported if taken in too high a dose. When taken in therapeutic doses in a two-weeks on, two-weeks off cycle, side-effects should not be a problem. It is best to avoid taking other stimulants such as caffeine containing products and drinks while taking ginseng.

Green Tea Extracts

Green and black tea are similar in that both are made from the young leaves and leaf buds of the same shrub, *Camellia sinensis*. Green tea is made by steaming and drying fresh tea leaves immediately after harvesting, while black tea is made by crushing and fermenting freshly cut tea leaves so they oxidize before drying. This allows natural enzymes in the tea leaves to produce the characteristic red-brown colour and reduced astringency.

Over 30 per cent of the dry weight of green tea leaves consists of powerful flavonoid antioxidants such as catechins, which are at least 100 times more powerful than vitamin C, and 25 times more powerful than vitamin E. These are converted into less active antioxidants (e.g. theaflavins and thearubigins) during fermentation, but still provide a significant antioxidant action. Research suggests that drinking either type of tea has beneficial effects on blood lipids, blood pressure, blood stickiness and can decrease the risk of coronary heart disease and stroke.

Antioxidants found in green tea extracts are also known to increase resistance to infection, and to protect against premature ageing.

Dose: Drink four cups of green tea daily, or take supplements: 500 mg daily (standardized to contain at least 50 per cent polyphenols).

Horsetail (Equisetum arvense)

Horsetail is an ancient plant related to trees growing on the earth 270 million years ago. It has brittle, jointed stems which when dried are mildly diuretic and can help to reduce pre-menstrual bloating associated with menopausal symptoms. It also tones the urinary tract and can help to reduce the embarrassing effects of stress incontinence as well as reducing fluid retention. One of its most useful actions for menopausal women is that it stops excessive sweating and is therefore a useful treatment for hot flushes and night sweats. Horsetail is also used to:

- staunch bleeding and hasten wound healing
- reduce blood loss in heavy periods
- improve the circulation
- treat skin conditions
- increase urinary flow and reduce urinary infection
- control bed-wetting
- improve the strength of dry, brittle nails due to its rich content of silica.

Dose: 1 g up to 3 times daily.

Japanese Arrowroot/Kudzu (Pueraria lobata)

Japanese Arrowroot is an Asian vine used as a traditional Chinese food. Its starchy root is used in soups and stews as a thickening agent similar to cornstarch. It contains beneficial plant hormones (betasitosterol and isoflavones such as daidzein and formononetin) similar to those found in soy, plus other unique isoflavones such as puerarin.

Kudzu is used as a source of isoflavones to reduce

menopausal symptoms of hot flushes and night sweats. It also appears to be effective in decreasing alcohol cravings.

Dose: 150 mg 3 times a day.

Liquorice (Glycyrrhiza glabra)

Liquorice rhizome contains a substance known as glycyrrhizin, which is 50 times sweeter than sucrose. Liquorice root also contains phytoestrogens and has a weak oestrogen like action similar to that of isoflavones. It helps to boost a low oestrogen state after the menopause, but its use is limited by potential side-effects.

Dose: 4 to 15 g per day of cut or powdered root. Extracts: 200 to 600 mg daily (standardized to 22 per cent glycyrrhizin).

Note: Liquorice that has not been deglycyrrhizinated can cause sodium retention if taken regularly in high doses. Glycyrrhizin intact liquorice needs to be stopped slowly rather than suddenly to prevent a rebound effect if used in high doses. It should not be used by people with liver disease, low potassium levels, kidney failure or high blood pressure, by those taking diuretics or digoxin, or during pregnancy. This form of liquorice should not be taken long term (e.g. for more than a month) except under supervision from a medical herbalist.

Maca (Lepidium meyenii)

Maca is a root vegetable, related to the potato, which grows in the Peruvian Andes. It is a good source of vitamins and minerals, and also contains a number of steroid glycosides with oestrogen-like actions. It helps to relieve menopausal symptoms and it is sometimes even referred to as Peruvian ginseng.

Dose: 1 g, 2 or 3 times a day.

Motherwort (Leonurus cardiaca)

The leaves of the motherwort plant have been used since Roman times to ease palpitations, regulate a fast pulse and to lower blood pressure. It is effective in relieving anxiety, and nervous tension around the time of the menopause and is also said to stimulate menstrual flow, ease period pains, and relieve hot flushes.

Dose: Up to 4 g daily.

Note: As it is a uterine stimulant, it is not usually advised during pregnancy (with the exception of labour).

Muira Puama (Ptychopetalum olacoides)

Muira Puama is a small Amazonian tree whose roots, bark and wood boost a low libido. It is thought to stimulate sexual desire through a direct action on brain chemicals, by stimulating nerve endings in the genitals and by boosting production/function of sex hormones, especially testosterone. A field trial involving 202 women suggested it is effective in around two out of three menopausal women who take it to counter a low sex drive at this time of life.

Dose: 1–1.5 g daily for two weeks.

Note: No serious side effects have been reported at therapeutic doses.

Oat Seed/Straw (Avena sativa)

Oat seeds are used as a tonic for the nervous system, especially when you are exhausted, feeling low, depressed or under stress. It is a useful source of B group vitamins, which are also needed in extra amounts during times of stress such as the menopause. As the entire plant (known as oatstraw) contains plant hormone building blocks, it is also used as a general aid for women suffering from oestrogen or thyroid deficiency. It also helps to reduce cravings and is helpful for those who are trying to stop smoking.

Dose: 1 dropperful fluid-extract or tincture 2 or 3 times daily.

Note: People who are sensitive to gluten (coeliac disease) should allow the tincture to settle, and decant the clear liquid for use.

Pfaffia (Pfaffia paniculata)

The dried root of Pfaffia – also known as Suma and Brazilian ginseng – contains a number of unique substances known as pfaffocides, plus phytoestrogens such as stigmasterol and sitosterol. Pfaffia is used to help normalize hormone imbalances such as pre-menstrual syndrome and menopausal symptoms, and can also boost physical, mental and sexual energy levels.

Dose: Extracts standardized to 5 per cent ecdysterones: 500 mg–1 gm daily to combat physical and mental stress. Larger doses of 15 a day are used in treating cancer.

Note: Diabetics should monitor sugar levels closely, as Pfaffia seems to boost insulin production, normalizes blood sugar levels and may reduce insulin requirements. Pfaffia should not be taken during pregnancy or breast-feeding. Pfaffia should not be taken by women with a history of endometriosis or female cancers, except under specialist advice.

Red Clover *(Trifolium pratense)*

Red Clover flowers contain three classes of oestrogen-like plant hormones, isoflavones, coumestans and lignans. It is one of the few plants to contain all four isoflavones – genistein, daidzein, formononetin (methoxy-daidzein) and biochanin A (methoxy-genistein) – which, plus other flavonoid glycosides, account for up to 2 per cent dry weight. It is widely used to provide an additional oestrogenic boost where oestrogen levels are low at the menopause. Studies have shown it can reduce menopausal symptoms of hot flushes and mood swings within three to four weeks as well as helping to produce increased energy levels and a more positive outlook on life. In one study, post-menopausal women taking Red Clover for two weeks and following an oestrogen-rich diet had significantly higher oestrogen levels, which then fell again when they stopped taking the supplements. Other studies have shown reduced menopausal symptoms of hot flushes and mood swings within three to four weeks of starting to take Red Clover, plus a more positive outlook on life and increased energy levels.

Dose: 500 mg tablet (standardized to contain 40mg isoflavones) daily.

Note: No serious side-effects have been reported. However, Red Clover should not be taken during pregnancy or while breast-feeding.

Soy Isoflavones

Soy contains plant hormones known as isoflavones, including genistein, daidzein, formononetin, biochanin A and glycitein. Isoflavones (See Chapter 9) have a weak, oestrogen-like action in the body, which is useful at the menopause as they can provide an additional oestrogen boost to help reduce symptoms of hot flushes and night sweats. Isoflavones act as a natural form of hormone replacement therapy.

A study involving over 100 post-menopausal women showed that isoflavones significantly reduced the number of hot flushes experienced per day. By the twelfth week of treatment, women taking soy had a 45 per cent reduction in hot flushes versus only 30 per cent with placebo.

Isoflavones also mimic the beneficial effects of oestrogen on bone, to boost formation of new bone and reducing absorption of old bone. A daily intake of 2.25 mg isoflavones has been shown to significantly increase bone mineral content and density in the lumbar spine and to protect against spinal bone loss and osteoporosis.

As an additional benefit, isoflavones appear to help reduce the risk of breast cancer. This effect is not yet fully understood but, as well as reducing the total amount of oestrogen stimulation the breasts receive (by blocking oestrogen receptors so that stronger human oestrogens cannot stimulate them), isoflavones reduce the activity of tumour growth factors in the laboratory, so that new blood vessels do not form in developing tumours and tumour cells fail to thrive. They also seem to protect genetic material from harmful mutations.

Dose: At least 2.25 to 50 mg isoflavones daily. 60 g of soy protein provides 45 mg isoflavones.

Note: There has been concern over a possible detrimental effect of isoflavone supplements in women with pre-existing breast cancer due to their oestrogen-like action. A recent review concluded that, overall, there is no impressive data suggesting that adult consumption of soy/isoflavones affects the risk of developing breast cancer or that soy consumption affects the survival of breast cancer patients. The review therefore concluded that, if women with breast cancer enjoy soy products, it seems reasonable for them to continue using them. The review included results of a recent, year-long study indicating that isoflavone supplements do not affect breast tissue density in pre-menopausal women and, in contrast to prescribed HRT, may decrease density in post-menopausal women. It also noted data suggesting that it is the progestogen component of HRT, not the oestrogen, that may increase the risk of developing breast cancer, and that there is no convincing evidence that HRT reduces survival in women with breast cancer.

However, women who have been diagnosed with breast cancer are often advised to avoid supplements containing isoflavones until clinical trials have shown they are beneficial in women with pre-existing disease.

Sage (Salvia officinalis)

Sage is a well-known culinary herb whose leaves are a popular herbal remedy for menopausal hot flushes and night sweats. Sage extracts were found in a clinical trial involving 39 women to decrease the frequency of hot flushes by 56 per cent over a period of eight weeks, versus a 5 per cent increase in frequency amongst those taking inactive placebo. Sage is said to improve memory and acts as a mental stimulant.

Dose: 2–5 ml tincture daily:

Note: As sage stimulates uterine contractions, it should be avoided during pregnancy, although small amounts are safe for use in cooking. It should not be used during breast-feeding unless its ability to dry up milk is required. It should be avoided by those with epilepsy.

Siberian Ginseng (Eleutherococcus senticosus)

The root of Siberian Ginseng contains substances known as eleutherosides that have a similar action to ginsenosides found in Korean ginseng, although the plants are not closely related.

Siberian Ginseng is an effective adaptogen, helping the body adapt and cope during times of stress. It is used extensively to improve stamina and strength, and has oestrogen-like activity that has been shown to relieve hot flushes, vaginal dryness, night sweats and anxiety.

Dose: 1–2 g per day. Choose a brand that is standardized to contain more than 1 per cent for eleutherosides. Start with a low dose in the morning at least 20 minutes before eating. If increasing the dose, work up slowly and take 2 or 3 times per day. Take on an empty stomach unless you find it too relaxing, in which case take it with meals.

Note: No serious side-effects have been reported. Do not use (except under medical advice) if you suffer from high blood pressure, a tendency to nose bleeds, heavy periods, insomnia, rapid heart beat (tachycardia), high fever or congestive heart failure. Do not take during pregnancy or when breast-feeding except under specific medical advice.

St John's Wort (Hypericum perforatum)

St John's Wort contains a number of unique substances such as hypericin, pseudohypericin and hyperforin that have an effective antidepressant action. It is thought to work mainly by prolonging the action of a brain neurotransmitter, serotonin, slowing its re-uptake once it has been released.

St John's Wort is as effective in treating mild to moderate depression as many antidepressant drugs, including imipramine and sertraline, lifting a low mood in at least two out of three people taking it. Studies involving over 5,000 people show that Hypericum can lift mild depression within two weeks of starting the course, with the optimum effect reached within six weeks. Three out of four people showed a marked improvement after only five weeks, with one in three becoming symptom-free.

St John's Wort can also increase a low sex drive in older women. Research involving 111 post-menopausal women (aged 45–65 years) with low sex drive plus physical exhaustion found that taking St John's Wort for three months helped 60 per cent became interested in sex again, to feel sexy and to enjoy or initiate sex with their partner. Eighty-two per cent also suffered less irritability, anxiety, low mood, hot flushes, sweating and disturbed sleep. Before the trial, 60 per cent said they were too exhausted for sex. At the end of the trial, none of them felt that way. They also reported increased self-esteem, a marked increase in self-confidence and self respect.

Dose: Extracts standardized to 0.3 per cent hypericin: 300 mg 3 times a day; 1-a-day formulas are also available.

Note: St John's Wort is best taken with food. Avoid alcohol when taking it, and it should not be taken during pregnancy or when breast-feeding. Avoid direct skin exposure to sunlight when taking it, especially if fair-skinned.

Do not take together with other antidepressants except under medical supervision. If taking other prescribed drugs, always check with a pharmacist to ensure there are no known interactions. Those currently recognized include interactions with warfarin, cyclosporin, oral contraceptives, anticonvulsants, digoxin, theophylline, HIV protease inhibitors and other antidepressants.

Despite this seemingly long list, St John's wort is a safe and effective treatment and when taken alone – and when combined with many drugs – it causes no harm. Side-effects are significantly less likely than with standard antidepressants. Those reported include indigestion allergic reactions, restlessness and tiredness/fatigue each in less than 1 per cent of people.

Valerian (Valerian officinalis)

Valerian roots contain substances (e.g. valeric acid, valepotriates) that help to make it one of the most calming herbs available. Its roots have been used since Mediaeval times to calm nervous anxiety, tension and to induce a refreshing night's sleep.

It helps to overcome low mood, loss of initiative, unsociability, irritability, anxiety and difficulty sleeping. A randomized, double-blind, placebo-controlled study involving 16 patients with primary insomnia found that 300 mg concentrated dry extract (equivalent to 1800 mg fresh herb) produced beneficial effects on slow wave sleep with, according to the researchers, 'an extremely low number of adverse events'.

Valerian is often used together with other calming herbs such as lemon balm and hops to ease nervous anxiety, insomnia and to help avoid a panic attack. It may also be used together with St John's Wort for depression.

Dose: 250–800 mg 2 to 3 times a day. Select standardized products containing at least 0.8 per cent valeric acid.

Note: Do not take if you are using prescribed sleeping tablets. Do not take during pregnancy or breast-feeding. It may cause mild drowsiness, which will affect your ability to drive or operate machinery.

Wild Yam (Dioscorea villosa)

Wild Yam is a Mexican vine whose root is rich in substances known as steroidal saponins, such as diosgenin. Diosgenin is a hormone-like substance originally used in the laboratory to synthesize a synthetic form of progesterone (norethisterone) used in the first oral contraceptive pills. Wild Yam cream sold as containing natural progesterone actually contains progesterone that has been synthetically produced in the laboratory from plant-like hormones found in Wild Yam. It is therefore a form of hormone replacement therapy, not a herbal remedy. The progesterone in these creams is synthetic, in that it is made in the laboratory and is only described as 'natural' as it has the same chemical structure as progesterone naturally found in the human body.

When applied to the skin, only small increases in

circulating progesterone levels are seen, as the hormone tends to accumulate in subcutaneous fat cells; even so, many women seem to find the creams helpful. In one study of 102 women, 83 per cent using progesterone cream for one year reported improvements in hot flushes, compared with only 19 per cent on placebo.

Wild Yam acts as a general tonic and is also used to help relieve painful periods.

Dose: Capsules: 250–500 mg once or twice a day.

Note: Excess may cause nausea or diarrhoea.

It should not be taken in pregnancy, except under medical supervision.

10
Weight and the Menopause

From middle age onwards, your metabolism starts to slow, by as much as 3 per cent per year, and activity levels tend to reduce, so there is a natural tendency to put on weight. Between the ages of 27 and 47, your metabolic rate may fall by 12 per cent – this means you need to cut back on the number of calories you eat, and increase your level of physical activity to avoid putting on weight. In practice, this often doesn't happen and the waistline begins to spread. Between the ages of 25 and 70, the average woman:

- increases her body fat percentage from 27 per cent to 40 per cent
- loses 5 kg of lean body mass (muscle) which falls from an average of 40 kg to 35 kg

By the age of 75, a woman needs around 300 kcals less per day than when she was 18, and 130 kcals per day less than when she was 50. If exercise levels remain the same, your calorie intake must drop to avoid putting on weight. As a rough guide, you need to eat 50 kcals per day less for every five years after the age of 27.

Falling levels of female sex hormones also mean you start to store excess fat differently than when you were younger. Rather than gaining weight on your breasts, hips and thighs for example, you may develop a more male pattern of weight gain, putting on weight around your abdomen.

Overweight increases the risk of serious diseases and premature death in post-menopausal women. Those who are overweight are one and a half times more likely to have a heart attack than someone who maintains a healthy weight, while those who are obese are at least twice as likely to die from weight-related conditions.

Are you Overweight?

Body fat stores are estimated using the Body Mass Index (BMI). This is calculated by dividing your weight in kilograms by your height in metres squared:

$$BMI = \frac{Weight\ (Kg)}{Height\ (M) \times Height\ (M).}$$

This gives a figure which is interpreted as follows:

<20	Underweight
20–25	Healthy weight
25–30	Overweight
30–40	Obese
>40	Morbidly Obese

The BMI calculation is only occasionally misleading. For

example, body builders with unusual high muscle mass may have a BMI of up to 30 without being obese. For women, however, who naturally have a greater fat percentage, slightly stricter BMI ranges apply for the healthy weight range based on a BMI of 18.7–23.8. To make this as easy as possible, the following chart shows the healthy weight range for height that you should aim for (based on BMI 18.7–23.8).

Height		Optimum Healthy Weight Range for Women	
Metres	Feet	Kg	Stones
1.47	4'10"	40–51	6st 4–8st
1.50	4'11"	42–54	6st 8–8st 7
1.52	5ft	43–55	6st 11–8st 9
1.55	5'1"	45–57	7st 1–8st 13
1.57	5'2"	46–59	7st 3–9st 4
1.60	5'3"	48–61	7st 8–9st 8
1.63	5'4"	50–63	7st 12–9st 13
1.65	5'5"	51–65	8st–10st 3
1.68	5'6"	53–67	8st 5–10st 7
1.70	5'7"	54–69	8st 7–10st 12
1.73	5'8"	56–71	8st 11–11st 2
1.75	5'9"	57–73	8st 13–11st 7
1.78	5'10"	59–75	9st 4–11st 11
1.80	5'11"	61–77	9st 8–12st 1
1.83	6 ft	63–80	9st 13–12st 8

Apples versus Pears

Where excess weight is stored is also important. If you are overweight and store fat round your middle (apple-shaped), you are twice as likely to develop coronary heart disease –

especially if this runs in your family. People who are apple-shaped have a higher risk of hardening and furring up of the arteries, high cholesterol levels, high blood pressure, coronary heart disease, stroke and diabetes than those who are pear-shaped. The reason is not fully understood, but is probably linked with the way your body handles dietary fats. Lack of exercise and drinking excessive amounts of alcohol also seem to encourage fat gain around the waist.

In fact, waist size alone may be a good indicator of health – or lack of it. Research suggests that women with a waist circumference larger than 88 cm are more likely to develop shortness of breath, high blood pressure, high cholesterol levels and diabetes than those with slimmer waistlines.

If you fall into this pattern of weight gain after the menopause, it is important to follow a low-fat diet and increase the amount of exercise you take. Slight waist reductions of just 5–10 cm significantly reduce the risk of having a heart attack. Getting down to the healthy weight range for your height can reduce your risk of a heart attack by as much as 35–55 per cent.

Is Overweight Hereditary?

Obesity develops due to a number of different factors working together, including the amount you eat, the amount of exercise you take and the genes you have inherited. Your genes help to control your metabolic rate and how efficiently you convert excess energy to body fat stores. Family eating habits and activity behaviour are also important. If both your parents are obese, you have a 70 per cent chance of obesity too, compared with less than 20 per cent if both your parents are lean.

Hormone problems are often blamed for overweight. Although these problems are uncommon, an underactive thyroid gland (hypothyroidism), or an overactive adrenal gland (Cushing's syndrome) may play a role in some cases, although they are not a common cause of obesity. If you are worried you may have a hormone problem, ask your doctor's advice. Most cases of obesity linked to hormone imbalances are quickly diagnosed and treatment can help to correct the problem.

Losing Excess Weight

The only way to lose weight is to eat fewer calories than you burn. It's best to do this slowly, at a rate of around 0.5–1 kg (1–2 lbs) weight loss per week. If you lose weight more rapidly than this, two undesirable things will happen: you will lose a greater percentage of lean tissue mass (muscle); and your metabolism will go onto red alert and become more efficient so less energy is wasted as heat and weight loss will slow.

As soon as you start eating more, your body fat stores will pile back on again – but not the muscle you lost. You may end up weighing more, but with less of that weight composed of muscle, than before you decided to diet. The best way to lose weight permanently is to change your eating habits, so you eat more healthily without feeling you're actually on a diet, and to increase the amount of exercise you take. Look on it as a healthy eating plan for the rest of your life, rather than a temporary slimming diet. The most important change is to cut back on your intake of dietary fats, which provide twice as many calories as carbohydrates (starch) and proteins per gram. See Chapter 8: Diet and the Menopause, for advice on healthy eating.

How much Exercise do you Need?

Exercise is the most effective way known to increase your metabolic rate (as much as ten-fold), mobilize fatty acids from fat cells and increase the burning of fatty acids as fuel in muscle cells. Research has also shown that when you indulge in prolonged brisk walking, your blood fat levels will rise much less than usual after eating, as dietary fats are rapidly burned for fuel rather than added to fat stores. This effect was noticed when exercise was taken as much as 15 hours before a meal, and when exercise was taken 90 minutes after a meal.

Exercise is an especially effective way to shift a spare tyre round your middle – however long it's been there. In one study, nearly 100 non-smoking volunteers aged 60–70, who had not exercised for at least two years, were started on a gentle programme of jogging, rowing or cycling for 45 minutes, three days a week. After a year, their body weight had not changed dramatically, as they had replaced flab with muscle (which is more dense). They had preferentially lost fat from around their middle, however, to lose their apple shape and had a slimmer silhouette.

Another study showed that following a two-month walking programme, in which you build up from two 15-minute sessions a week to a total of two hours per week, can take a total of four inches off your waist, hips and thighs even if you keep eating the same amount.

You will find information on different forms of exercise in the next chapter.

Anti-obesity Drugs

Some people who are obese may benefit from prescribed drugs, either to reduce the amount of fat absorbed from their diet or to reduce their appetite. Currently, only two 'slimming' drugs are available on prescription for people who meet strict criteria. A prescription-only drug, orlistat, works by blocking the action of digestive enzymes, known as lipases, to reduce the absorption of dietary fat by an average of 30 per cent. Trials show that overweight people taking orlistat can lose nearly twice as much weight, and maintain that weight loss over two years, compared with those following a diet alone. Almost half maintained a weight loss above 10 per cent after one year. For someone weighing 100 kg (15 st 10 lb), this represents a weight loss of 10 kg (1 st 8 lb) body fat, which can significantly improve obesity-related conditions such as high blood pressure, abnormally raised blood fat levels, and raised blood glucose levels. Orlistat is taken before, during or up to one hour after each main meal (up to three times a day) and is prescribed together with a weight management programme which includes a low-fat diet. It is only licensed for use in those who are clinically obese (or who are overweight with other risk factors for coronary heart disease) who have been able to lose more than 2.5 kg in weight over a period of 4 weeks, using diet alone.

Sibutramine affects the levels of chemicals in the brain to make you feel fuller quicker and reduce appetite so you eat less. In trials with sibutramine, 90 per cent of people who responded during the first four weeks of treatment went on to lose over a stone in weight (7.7 kg) by the end of a year. In comparison, of those receiving inactive placebos only 61 per cent managed to lose 2.4 kg after 12 months treatment.

If you are obese, your doctor can advise whether or not drug treatment is likely to help you lose weight combined with a sensible diet and lifestyle changes.

Weight Loss Supplements

Some weight loss supplements may be helpful in curbing appetite and speeding fat loss when combined with a sensible diet and exercise regime.

GUARANA

Herbal extracts from three Amazonian plants: guarana, damiana and yerba mate (sold as Zotrim) slow the rate of stomach emptying to help reduce food intake, and help you feel full, faster and for longer. In a recent clinical study, 47 overweight people were divided into two groups. Those who took Zotrim lost an average of 11 lb over 45 days, compared with under 1 lb in those taking placebo.

CONJUGATED LINOLEIC ACID

Conjugated linoleic acid (CLA) is a fatty acid mainly found in meat and dairy products. Commercially, it is synthesized from sunflower and safflower oils. CLA cannot be synthesized in the human body and the average diet only supplies up to 300 mcg CLA daily, while our ancestors obtained a more optimum 3000 mg. It is often referred to as the 'missing link' in weight loss management, and some researchers even claim obesity is a CLA deficiency disease. CLA regulates enzymes involved in the mobilization and transport of dietary fats so that less fat is laid down in fatty tissues, and more fat is transported to muscle cells – building muscle at the expense of fat.

In one study, ten volunteers took 3 g CLA daily, and another group of ten subjects took placebo. After three months, those taking CLA had only lost around 2 lbs in weight (156.6 lb down to 154.4 lb), but their body fat percentage fell significantly from 21.3 per cent to 17 per cent. Those taking placebo gained half a pound in weight and their body fat percentage increased slightly from 22 per cent to 22.4 per cent.

Because it affects the body's ratio of lean to fatty tissue, people taking it often experience a reduction in waist size (average loss of 1.6 inches in one study), even when they do not make any other changes to their diet or lifestyle.

CLA may be most helpful as a weight management aid rather than a weight loss aid. It may also have beneficial actions against coronary heart disease by reducing blood triglyceride and cholesterol levels.

CHITOSAN

One of the main causes of obesity is eating too much fat which, gram for gram, contains twice as many calories as carbohydrate or protein. Chitosan is a fibre supplement derived from shellfish, which aids weight loss by absorbing dietary fat in the intestines so that less is absorbed and more is excreted. This helps you maintain a low fat intake and can also reduce circulating blood fat levels.

In a number of randomized clinical trials with volunteers following a low-calorie diet, those taking chitosan experienced significantly more weight loss than those taking placebo over a four-week period. In one trial of 100 overweight or obese volunteers who followed a low-calorie diet, those taking chitosan supplements for four weeks lost 7.3 kg compared with 3 kg in those taking placebo.

HYDROXYCITRIC ACID

Hydroxycitric acid (HCA) is a fruit acid originally derived from the rind of an exotic fruit, Garcinia cambogia. HCA is related to citric acid and is believed to block a metabolic enzyme responsible for converting excess dietary carbohydrate and protein into fat. Excess carbohydrate is diverted into the production of glycogen – a starchy, muscle energy store – instead. It also curbs the appetite.

In a placebo-controlled study, 50 overweight adults took either HCA (NatraShape in varying doses) or placebo, and were instructed not to change their normal dietary lifestyle. After four weeks, the body weight of those in the placebo group had increased by an average of 1.3 kg, while those taking HCA had reduced by between 2.2 kg and 5.5 kg, directly related to the daily dose of HCA taken. Subjective evaluation of appetite levels showed considerable reduction in those taking HCA, but not in the placebo group.

Chewing gum containing HCA plus chromium is useful for stopping snacking between meals (especially in those who are quitting smoking) as well as helping to reduce intake at meal times.

IODINE CONTAINING SUPPLEMENTS

Iodine is essential for the production of thyroxine, a hormone that regulates metabolism. The normal range for thyroxine hormone is wide, with the upper limit of normal three times greater than the lower. If iodine intakes are low (sources include iodized salt, seaweed and seafood) thyroxine levels may be in the lower normal range. Supplements providing iodine act as a mild thyroid stimulant and may encourage a more efficient metabolism if your iodine intake has been sub-optimal. Iodine may also improve energy levels and quality of skin, hair and nails.

Note: Not suitable for those with thyroid problems (except under medical advice).

CHROMIUM

Trivalent chromium is needed in minute amounts to form an organic complex known as Glucose Tolerance Factor (GTF). GTF encourages the production of energy from glucose, and lowers blood fat levels, including harmful LDL cholesterol. It may also suppress hunger pangs through a direct effect on the satiety centre in the brain. Chromium deficiency is common and may affect as many as 90 per cent of adults. Low levels of chromium have been linked with poor glucose tolerance and diabetes, hunger pangs and weight gain.

In one study, 233 people randomly received placebo or chromium for 72 days, without receiving weight loss, dietary or exercise guidance – subjects could follow whichever type of weight loss programme they wished. Statistical analysis showed that those receiving placebo had an average body weight of 83.3 kg before the trial, and only lost 0.4 kg over the 72 days. Those receiving chromium picolinate (at least 200 mg) had an initial weight of 84.6 kg and lost an average of 1.26 kg. There were also significant improvements in body composition (more fat lost, compared with lean tissue).

GREEN TEA EXTRACTS

An extract from green tea leaves (*Camellia sinensis*) known as AR 25 catechol (sold as Exolize) has been shown in clinical studies with healthy volunteers to boost the rate at which the body burns calories by as much as 40 per cent over a 24 hour period. This is due to its ability to inhibit a metabolic enzyme (catechol methyl transferase) so that levels of noradrenaline increase to stimulate the amount of energy burned in body cells (thermogenesis). It also blocks the activity of intestinal enzymes (gastric and pancreatic lipases) needed to digest dietary fat, so that 30 per cent less fat is absorbed overall. Clinical trials involving 80 overweight men and women who took green tea extracts found they lost 3.5 kg over three months, with a decrease in waist circumference of 1 cm.

CoQ10

The vitamin-like Co-enzyme Q10 (CoQ10), also known as ubiquinone, is an essential component of the mitochondria in the energy producing unit of the cells of our body. Lack of CoQ10 becomes increasingly common with age and contributes to a number of ageing conditions, including weight gain. Supplements may be useful in weight loss by stimulating lipid metabolism in mitochondria. A pilot study found that nine obese subjects (average age 37 years) who were deficient in CoQ10 were placed on a weight loss diet; those taking 100 mg CoQ10 daily lost an average of 30 lbs compared with an average of 13 lbs for those not taking CoQ10. See Chapter 9: Nutritional Supplements and their Benefits, for further information on CoQ10.

AROMATHERAPY

The desire for food is often stimulated by your sense of smell and conversely, certain scents can be used to overwhelm your sense of smell and reduce your desire to taste food. Inhaling Banana, Green Apple or Peppermint essences on alternating days can help reduce food cravings so you eat less overall. Inhaling vanilla scents can help you overcome cravings for chocolate.

11
Exercise and Lifestyle

By the time you reach the menopause, your body will have started to change in a number of ways and once oestrogen levels fall, these changes accelerate, so that between the ages of 30 and 70, your:

- lean body tissue (muscle) will have decreased from an average of 40 to 35 kg
- metabolic rate will have slowed by around 5 per cent every ten years
- body fat percentage will have increased from 27 per cent to 40 per cent of body weight
- excess body fat will be stored more around your middle so you become increasingly apple-rather than pear-shaped (see Chapter 9)
- suppleness will decrease as joints, ligaments and muscles become less flexible.

Also, after the menopause, your:

- bone density will fall by an average of 2–3 per cent per year
- your strength will reduce by around 1–2 per cent per year
- your power (strength multiplied by speed) will reduce by 3–4 per cent per year.

Exercise

The changes outlined above occur slowly and subtly, but add up to produce significant changes to health over time. Exercise can help to postpone these effects of ageing, however, and can even prolong your life – even if it is not started until middle age. In the over 45s, exercise has been shown to help you:

- feel more energized
- fell less anxious and stressed
- sleep better
- reduce abdominal fat storage so you become less apple-shaped
- improve your strength, stamina and suppleness
- maintain a healthy weight
- reduce high blood cholesterol levels
- reduce your risk of high blood pressure by 40 per cent
- reduce your risk of a heart attack by over 40 per cent
- reduce your risk of stroke by 33 per cent
- reduce the risk of diabetes by 29 per cent
- stimulate formation of new bone to reduce your risk of a hip fracture by 60 per cent.
- keep your bowels regular.

Unfortunately, eight out of ten women do not take enough exercise to reduce their risk of heart disease or benefit from many of the other protective effects. Even if you have not exercised much before, it is not too late to start NOW.

How Much Exercise do I Need?

If you can exercise moderately for 30 minutes, at least five times per week – and preferably every day – you can halve your risk of a heart attack compared with someone who is physically inactive. And you don't have to become an exercise freak – the good news is that activities such as DIY, gardening and dancing are just as effective as swimming or cycling for heart health. Any activity that leaves you feeling warm and slightly out of breath is doing you good. Researchers have also found that your half hour of exercise doesn't have to be completed all in one go – you can divide it into two or three daily sessions of 10–15 minutes if you prefer.

Your exercise needs to be brisk enough to raise your pulse above 100 beats per minute, raise a light sweat and make you slightly breathless – but not so much that you cannot hold a conversation.

What Types of Exercise Should I Choose?

Several different aspects of exercise are important at this time of life. Regular stretch exercises will help to keep your muscles and joints supple, while for a beneficial effect on heart and lung fitness, you also need to build cardiovascular exercises such as brisk walking, hill walking, cycling, swimming, rowing or gentle jogging into your regime – most of which will benefit your bones and other aspects of health, too. Regular exercise that is weight bearing and increases muscle strength is known to protect against osteoporosis by boosting the production of new bone. As well as stimulating blood circulation and increasing the supply of minerals to the bones, it also activates the bone network of cells to encourage strengthening in areas of high stress and weakness. See pages 205–216 for more on appropriate forms of exercise.

Exercise and Osteoporosis

Surprisingly, bones respond to mechanical pressures applied to them, so that areas under stress become thicker and stronger. Bones are not just dry sticks, but contain millions of tiny spaces in which lie a network of cells that connect with each other through fine strands of tissue. When bone is stressed, these strands are also stretched, pulled, compressed and twisted, which acts as a signal to stimulate production of new bone in these areas. As a result, bone density increases locally at the sites where bone is under greatest stress. Daily weight bearing exercise therefore helps to build up your bones and prevent osteoporosis by putting pressure on your bones as well as by increasing muscle strength. The forces that act on your bones to stimulate thickening include:

- traction which stretches the bone
- compression that squashes the bone
- bending which flexes the bone
- torsion which twists the bone.

Exercise also stimulates blood circulation so that more oxygen and nutrients such as calcium reach your bones.

By strengthening your muscles and improving your stamina, suppleness and balance, regular exercise also reduces the likelihood of a fall in older people. Together with the bone strengthening effect of exercise, this decreases the risk of sustaining an osteoporotic bone fracture. Studies have shown that exercise strengthens bone in pre-menopausal and post-menopausal women and in men. For example, when a group of post-menopausal women started an exercise regime consisting of five to ten minutes stretching followed by 30 minutes walking, jogging or dancing three times a week for a year, their bones were found to be significantly stronger than in a similar group of women who did not exercise.

In contrast, physical inactivity greatly increases the chance of a hip fracture, as can immobility (e.g. through wearing a plaster cast or being bedridden) as it leads to reduced mechanical stress on bones, and increased bone thinning. In one study, a group of women aged 53–74 years with mild osteoporosis were given bone-loading exercises to perform for 50 minutes, three times a week. Over the course of a year, their bone density increased by 4 per cent. A similar group of women who did not do these exercises continued to lose bone at a rate of up to 3 per cent over the same period – resulting in a 7 per cent benefit from exercising overall. If exercise stops, however, bone mass will slowly fall again, so it is important to maintain your level of physical activity for sustained benefit. Luckily, these bone-thinning effects of lack of exercise are reversible and starting a regular exercise regime can help to re-strengthen bones and reduce the risk of osteoporosis, even in later life.

Weight-bearing activities that stress your bones in all these ways are most beneficial for strengthening them. These are generally high impact in nature such as:

- aerobics
- gymnastics
- netball
- dancing
- racquet sports
- jogging
- running
- skipping.

Research in which women aged 35–45 years regularly took part in high impact exercise (jumping or step aerobics) for 18 months showed that their bone mineral density increased by a massive 14 per cent to 37 per cent. This type of regular activity requires a high degree of commitment to reap the benefits, however. It is best to choose an activity that you enjoy and which you are likely to continue, than to start a demanding regime that you are unlikely to keep up.

Non-weight-bearing exercises such as swimming can also have a beneficial effect on bone, as the muscle movements that bend your joints and flex your back also stress your bones slightly. Swimming is especially appropriate if you have problems with your joints, such as arthritis. Stretching exercises can also be very beneficial – try following the programme suggested below.

STRETCH EXERCISES FOR BONES AND JOINTS

The following stretch exercises will help to improve your joint mobility, strengthen your muscles and bones and reduce your risk of osteoporosis. Repeat them at least five to ten times, once or twice a day:

Neck stretch: Stand comfortably with feet apart and shoulders relaxed. Slowly drop your left ear towards your left shoulder and hold the stretch for a count of five. Repeat on the right hand side.

Shoulders: Stand comfortably, with feet apart. Bend your arms up and clasp your hands behind your head. Pull your elbows forward so they almost touch in front of your chin, then swing your elbows out so they are as wide apart as possible.

Put your arms up behind your back as if trying to fasten your bra (or if you prefer, putting your hands in your back pockets) then lower them again.

Raise your arms above your head, keeping them straight, and stretch as high as you can.

Raise one arm out to your side and slowly swing it around to make a big circle.

Arms: Stand facing a wall, two feet away, with your feet a hip-width apart. Keep your back straight, your abdominal muscles pulled in and your pelvis tilted forward. Place your hands flat on the wall, in line with your shoulders, with your fingers pointing up. Do 'push ups' by bending your elbows and leaning in so your nose almost touches the wall – keep your back flat and legs straight. Hold this position briefly, then use your arms to push away from the wall. (Breathe in as you bend in, breathe out as you push out).

Wrists: Bend both wrists up and down, side to side and round and round as far as possible.

Fingers: Squeeze a soft foam ball in the palm of your hand by clenching your fingers as tightly as possible. Hold for a count of five, then relax and strengthen your fingers.

Pelvis: Lie on the floor, or a firm mattress. Bend your knees up, and place your feet flat on the floor and relax your arms on the floor above your head. Now tighten the muscles of your lower abdomen and buttocks, so your pelvis tilts and the small of your back flattens against the floor. Hold for a count of five, then relax and repeat.

Hips: Stand comfortably with feet apart and hands on your hips. Without moving your lower body, rotate your upper body and hips to the right, to the back, to the left and to the front again. Repeat 5 times in one direction, then 5 times in the other.

Lie on the floor, with both legs bent so your feet are flat on the floor. Lift one leg up into the air and straighten it. Hold for a count of five. Repeat with the other leg. (*Note*: When straightening one leg, always keep the other knee bent to protect your back. Don't try to lift both legs into the air at the same time.)

Legs: Stand comfortably with your back and head straight, tummy tucked in and feet apart. Rest your left hand on a table for support. Bend your left knee slightly, and raise your right leg to grasp your right ankle with your right hand. Keep your knees facing forward. Gently ease your foot in towards your bottom until you feel a mild stretch. Hold for a count of five. Repeat with the other side.

Stand with your back two feet away from a wall, your feet a hip-width apart and your toes pointing forwards. Pull in your abdominal muscles, relax your shoulders, and bend your knees and hips to around 90 degrees, pressing your lower back into the wall. Hold this position for at least 50 seconds.

Stand comfortably with feet apart, knees bent and hands

on your knees. Flex your knees up and down, keeping them bent throughout. Don't let your bottom go lower than the level of your knees.

Ankles: Stand comfortably, resting one hand on a table for support. Lift one foot and rotate the ankle in ten complete circles, first clockwise, then anticlockwise. Repeat with the other foot.

Stand comfortably, feet slightly apart, with one hand resting on a table for support. Lift both heels up so you are stand on the ball of your foot, then relax down again.

Choosing the Right Form of Exercise

Different types of exercise have different effects on your strength, stamina, suppleness and bone density:

Activity	Strength	Stamina	Suppleness	Bone Density
Aerobics	**	***	***	****
Athletics	***	***	**	****
Badminton	**	**	***	****
Circuit Training	***	***	***	***
Cricket	*	*	**	***
Cycling	***	****	**	*
Dancing	**	****	***	****
Football	***	***	***	***
Jogging	**	****	**	****
Netball	***	****	***	****
Skipping	**	***	**	****
Squash	**	***	***	****
Swimming (hard)	****	****	****	*
Tennis	**	**	***	****

Activity	Strength	Stamina	Suppleness	Bone Density
Walking (brisk/hill)	**	***	*	**
Yoga	*	*	***	*

* = Slight effect   *** = Very good effect
** = Beneficial effect   **** = Excellent effect

Choose an Activity to Suit you

Most people give up exercise within a week or so because they don't enjoy it, find it boring, or because they have started off too quickly and felt tired, stiff, or uncomfortable. You are more likely to continue with a regular exercise regime if you tailor it to your individual needs.

If you prefer exercising alone, choose:

- Walking — especially brisk or hill walking
- Cycling
- Swimming
- A home gym work-out
- Jogging
- Gardening.

If you prefer companionable exercise, choose:

- walking a dog
- golf
- bowling
- table tennis
- work-out at a sports gym
- aerobic class
- dancing class

- keep-fit class
- tennis or badminton
- rambling club
- synchronized swimming club
- team sport such as netball, volleyball, ladies football, rounders, cricket or hockey.

If you need motivation or someone to direct you, think about investing in a:

- home exercise video
- personal trainer
- aerobic class
- exercise class at a sports centre
- exercise organized by a club.

Choose a Time to Suit You

It is important that your chosen form of exercise can fit into your daily routine for you to have any hope of keeping it up. This may be:

- early morning before setting off for work
- on your way to or from work (e.g. walking part of the way)
- in your lunch hour
- after work
- in the early evening.

Bear in mind that it is a good idea to do only light exercise – such as walking round the block with the dog – before going to bed, otherwise it may interfere with sleep.

Start Gently

If you are relatively unfit, don't launch straight into a hard fitness programme. Start off slowly and take regular exercise lasting at least 20 minutes, for a minimum of three times per week. Slowly build up time and effort you spend on exercise and once you have achieved a reasonable level of fitness, aim to do more.

Remember

- Always warm up first with a few simple bends and stretches
- Cool down afterwards by walking slowly for a few minutes
- Wear loose clothing and proper footwear specifically designed for the job and use any recommended safety equipment
- Don't exercise straight after a heavy meal, after drinking alcohol or if you feel unwell
- Stop immediately if you feel dizzy, faint, unusually short of breath or develop chest pain.

Note: If you are under your doctor's care for any condition – especially a heart problem – or are taking medication, seek medical advice before starting a physical exercise programme.

Using Your Pulse Rate

Measuring your pulse rate during exercise will ensure you stay within the safe range for burning excess fat and improving cardiovascular fitness without over-stressing your heart. Your pulse is most easily felt on the inner side of your wrist on the same side as your thumb (radial pulse) and at the side of the neck, under the jaw (carotid pulse).

Take your ten-second pulse every ten minutes or so during your exercise period, and make sure it stays within the ten-second pulse range for your age, as shown on the following chart:

AGE	10 Second Pulse Range
20–29	20–27
30–39	19–25
40–49	18–23
50–59	17–22
60–69	16–21
70 +	15–20

If you are unfit, make sure your pulse stays at the lower end of your ten-second pulse range at first, and slowly work up towards the upper end of the range for your age over several weeks.

If at any time your pulse rate goes higher than it should, stop exercising and walk around slowly until your pulse falls. When you restart, take things a little more easy. At the end of 20 minutes exercise, you should feel invigorated rather than exhausted. Stop if at any time you develop pain, become so breathless you can't speak, develop chest tightness or pain, feel dizzy or unwell and seek medical advice if appropriate.

Try taking your pulse one minute after stopping exercise, too. The more rapidly your pulse rate falls, the fitter you are. After ten minutes rest, your heart rate should fall to below 100 beats per minute. If you are very fit, your pulse will drop by up to 70 beats in one minute.

Vary Your Routine

It is worth changing your exercise routine regularly – perhaps every six months, in fact. Research shows that in women aged over 55 (i.e. post-menopausal) bone density peaked around six months after starting a regular exercise regime such as weight training or aerobics, but that this benefit was lost after a year. Therefore, if you continue to exercise in the same way, all you are doing is maintaining bone mass (which is better than not exercising, when bone mass would fall) rather than building new bone and increasing bone density. By changing the type of exercise you do, your bones will experience new stresses in different areas that continue the bone building process for optimum effect.

Tips to Help you Exercise More

1. Take up an active hobby such as ballroom dancing, bowls, swimming, golf, walking or cycling.
2. If you dislike exercise, try to put more effort into DIY or gardening.
3. Spend less time watching TV and more time pottering in the garden or around the house – listen to music or the radio if you like background noise.
4. Borrow a dog and take it for regular walks.
5. Walk up stairs rather than using the lift or escalator.
6. Walk or cycle reasonable distances rather than taking the car.
7. Try to take a short walk at least once a day (e.g. walk around the block in your lunch hour).
8. Walk briskly rather than dawdling whenever possible.
9. If you can't go out, try walking up and down stairs a few times a day.
10. Re-introduce the traditional habit of a family walk after the Sunday roast.
11. Get off the bus or tube one stop earlier than usual and walk the rest of the way.
12. Start getting up an hour earlier than usual and go for a

walk, cycle, do some gardening, fetch the daily paper, or visit the gym
13. Buy a home exercise machine and use it while watching the evening news.
14. Buy an exercise video and follow the routine regularly.

Lifestyle

As well as exercise, several other aspects of your lifestyle can affect your long-term health after the menopause. These include smoking, alcohol intake, excess aluminium intake, stress levels, the amount of relaxation you get and the quality of your sleep.

Smoking

Smoking cigarettes significantly increases the risk of osteo-porosis by lowering blood oestrogen levels and it can trigger a premature menopause two to five years earlier than normal. Smoking also reduces the activity of bone-building cells (osteoblasts) so that less new bone is made.

Stopping smoking also has other major benefits in reducing risk of a variety of other diseases. Smokers are three times more likely to have a heart attack than non-smokers and nine out of ten cancers are linked to cigarettes. As a result, on average, non-smokers tend to live six years longer than smokers.

How to Stop Smoking
Nicotine is addictive and giving up smoking takes a lot of commitment. Your doctor or practice nurse can help you formulate a Quit plan. For example:

- name the day to give up and get into the right frame of mind beforehand
- throw away all your cigarettes and smoking equipment such as cigarette papers, matches, lighters and ashtrays
- take it one day at a time
- keep a chart and tick off each successful cigarette-free day
- take extra exercise which stimulates release of brain chemicals that help to curb nicotine cravings
- keep active with DIY jobs in the evening rather than sitting in front of the TV
- avoid situations where you used to smoke
- learn to say 'No thanks, I've given up', and mean it
- ask friends and relatives not to smoke around you
- Plan a reward for every week of cigarette-free success.

When you have an urge to smoke, try:

- sucking on an artificial cigarette or herbal stick available in chemist shops
- sucking on celery or carrot sticks
- eating an apple
- cleaning your teeth with strong flavoured toothpaste
- going out for a brisk walk, swim, cycle-ride or jog
- taking a supplement containing oat straw, which can reduce cravings.
- ask a pharmacist about aromatherapy devices that help reduce cravings and about nicotine replacement therapy, which can be highly successful in helping people quit.

If withdrawal symptoms are particularly strong, try the following breathing exercise to help reduce your stress levels:

- breathe in slowly and deeply

- when you reach your limit of breathing in, immediately start to breathe out – without holding your breath – to empty your lungs as much as possible
- repeat five times without holding your breath in between.

Alcohol

You will find information on the benefits of a moderate intake of alcohol in the chapter on diet. However, if you drink more than the recommended maximum, it is important that you cut back. Kudzu (Japanese arrowroot) is a traditional food substance that is used to help reduce alcohol intake in those who find this difficult. Studies have shown that daidzein and daidzin, two isoflavones extracted from kudzu root, could suppress ethanol intake in the Golden hamster, a species that would otherwise voluntarily increase intakes of alcohol and reduce intakes of water when given a free choice. The suppression of alcohol intake was similar to that seen when hamsters were tested with other anti-alcoholism drugs.

As a nutritional supplement with little risk of toxicity, and a traditional history of successful use in alcohol-dependent humans, it is well worth trying if you experience troublesome alcohol cravings.

Aluminium

Long-term exposure to aluminium increases your risk of osteoporosis by interfering with calcium absorption from the gut, reducing deposition of calcium in bone and reducing collagen formation to weaken the bone matrix. Ideally, you should also stop using aluminium saucepans, or at least avoid cooking acidic foods such as rhubarb in them. This is because such foods interact with the aluminium oxide on the surface of the pain to dissolve it (and make the pan go shiny). When rhubarb was cooked in a stainless steel pain, it contained 0.1 mg aluminium per portion. When cooked in an aluminium pan, it contained 250 times as much (25 mg per portion). You should also consider avoiding using aluminium-containing antacids if you suffer from indigestion or heartburn.

Stress

The amount of stress you are under can have a profound effect on the type of menopause you experience. Women who lead a demanding, stressful life seem more likely to suffer distressing menopausal symptoms – probably because they lose the additional back-up normally provided by the adrenal gland to offset the effects of failing ovaries.

WHAT IS STRESS?

Stress is a modern term that simply means you are experiencing an abnormal amount of pressure. A certain amount of pressure is essential to help you meet life's challenges, release your creativity and fuel your continued personal growth. Once pressure falls outside the range with which you feel comfortable, however, it can lead to the unpleasant physical and emotional symptoms associated with distress. Different people are comfortable with different amounts of pressure, and how you cope varies from person to person and even from time to time.

Pressure is so important for survival, that the body is programmed to produce a stress response known as the flight or fight reaction. It is this reaction – due mainly to the effects of adrenaline hormone – that produces most of the physical and emotional feelings you experience when distressed. If your body did not produce adrenaline, feelings of stress would not occur, but as you would not respond appropriately to the tasks and dangers of every day life, you would not last long in the urban jungles of modern life.

Adrenaline (epinephrine) is produced by the adrenal glands, of which there are two – one above each kidney. The outer regions (cortex) of these small, triangular shaped glands produce hormones that affect the metabolism while their inner parts – known as the medulla – from part of the body's sympathetic nervous system. This branch of the nervous system is designed to act as the body's first line of defence during times of stress.

When you are confronted with a stressful situation that may require increased physical activity, nerve signals from the brain trigger the release of adrenaline from the adrenal medulla directly into your bloodstream. As a result, stress increases blood levels of adrenaline by as much as 1,000-fold within just one minute. Adrenaline then produces an instant response in different parts of the body, so your whole system goes onto red alert.

Are You Suffering From Stress?
The physical symptoms of stress can include:

- tiredness
- sweating
- flushing
- nausea
- insomnia
- palpitations
- rapid pulse
- dizziness

- faintness
- trembling
- pins and needles
- numbness
- headache
- chest pain
- stomach pain
- diarrhoea
- period problems.

Emotional symptoms can include:

- loss of concentration
- being unable to make decisions
- a tendency to become vague and forgetful
- defensiveness and inability to take criticism
- extreme anger
- overwhelming feelings of anxiety and panic
- fear of failure or rejection
- feelings of guilt and shame
- negative thoughts
- moodiness
- loss of sex drive and sexual problems
- obsessive or compulsive behaviour
- feelings of isolation
- a feeling of impending doom.

The behavioural symptoms of stress can include:

- compulsive eating habits
- excessive use of alcohol or tobacco
- abuse of drugs
- avoidance of places or situations

- increased aggression
- change in sleeping habits, particularly early wakening.

Many of these stress-related symptoms are similar to those that occur as a result of the menopause, and it is sometimes difficult to untangle whether your problems are hormonal or stress-related.

POSITIVE PRESSURE VERSUS NEGATIVE STRESS

Short-term positive pressure is a healthy part of everyday life. It gives you the energy and reserves you need to rise to the challenges of life, helping you strive to achieve your best. By psyching yourself up and preparing physically and mentally for particular situations, positive pressure improves your performance and motivation so you are more likely to meet your goals. It also allows you to feel a wonderful glow of satisfaction when the pressure is over, the energy mobilized has been consumed, you have prevailed and your body powers back down to its normal settings.

Excessive or long-term pressure has a negative effect, however, and keeps the fight or flight reaction switched on to drain you of energy – especially if it is not accompanied with physical activity. This is best thought of as negative stress, to differentiate it from positive pressure. Negative stress is due to persistently high levels of adrenaline and can lead to stress-related problems such as tension headache, digestive disorders and muscular cramps. Ultimately it can also lead to depressed immunity, high blood pressure and other potentially serious health threats if the negative stress is not addressed.

HOW YOU RESPOND TO STRESSFUL SITUATIONS

Whether or not you feel positive pressure or negative stress in a particular situation depends largely on the way you respond psychologically to that situation or in other words, on the way you interact with your environment. This is known as the *interactional* model of stress, in which stress is thought to result from an imbalance between the demands being made on you (real or perceived) and your ability (real or perceived) to cope with them.

Some situations almost always cause stress for most people and are usually those that over-stimulate the senses such as excess noise, extreme heat or cold and extreme physical exertion. Lack of stimulation – i.e. boredom – can also be stressful.

The way you respond to stress depends on a wide range of factors, including your:

- Personal circumstances (e.g. how your love-life, finances and career are going)
- Natural talents (e.g. communication skills, intelligence, ability with numbers)
- Previous experiences and expectations (particularly of the currently stressful situation)
- Ability to recognize you are stressed and to quickly do something about it
- Self-esteem and perception of how you will cope
- Physical fitness
- Organizational and time management skills
- Personality traits
- Diet and how healthy it is
- Ability to relax.

COPING WITH STRESS

Everyone will feel stressed from time to time, whatever their lifestyle or age. Short-term stress is not harmful and if you use it positively it will help you out in a tricky situation. Challenges add zest to life and propel you on to greater achievements. Stress is only a problem when it makes you feel distressed. The key to successful stress management is to obtain the right balance between pressures you can handle and the overload that drags you down. In this respect, the crucial balance is not usually that between real-demands on you and your actual capability, but between the way you perceive these demands in relation to how you think you can cope. The power of mind over matter can sway the balance between successfully coping with a stressful situation and knowing you will fail before you've even begun.

Although your stress response is largely automatic, you can consciously exert some control over two of its main features – your pattern of breathing and the amount of tension building up in your muscles.

When the body powers down from a high pressure situation, the fight or flight response is switched off and an opposite reaction known as the rest and digest response is triggered. You can consciously help to switch off your stress response by altering your breathing pattern and by relaxing your muscles with a relaxation exercise. This starts to reverse some of the changes produced during the flight or fight reaction to stress, so that digestion restarts, your breathing and heartbeat slow down and the tension in your muscles slowly recedes.

Quick tips to stop stress in its tracks

- Stop what you are doing and inwardly say 'Calm' to yourself
- If you are sitting down, stand up and gently stretch to your fullest possible extent
- Take a deep breath in and let it out slowly, concentrating on the movement of your diaphragm. Do this two or three times until you start to feel more in control. One of the breathing exercises below may also help
- Shake your hands and arms briskly, then shrug your shoulders
- If possible, go for a brisk walk, even if it is only briefly around the room or to the bathroom, to help get your circulation going again
- If possible, go somewhere private and groan or shout as loudly as you can. This can be very therapeutic. Some people find it helpful to punch a soft cushion as hard as possible
- Place a few drops of the flower essence, Rescue Remedy, under your tongue
- Inhale a personally chosen blend of aromatherapy oils made by adding a total of 15 drops essential oils to 30 ml carrier oil. Select two or three oils to blend from: Bergamot, Cardamom, Camomile, Coriander, Geranium, Grapefruit, Lavender, Lemon, Neroli or Sandalwood.

ANXIETY AND PANIC ATTACKS

Anxiety is one of the main symptoms of stress and is associated with feelings of apprehension, dread, panic and impending doom. While short-lived anxiety is appropriate in some situations (e.g. when going for an interview) those with morbid anxiety worry excessively about trivial matters and frequently experience other typical stress symptoms such as restlessness, palpitations, tremor, flushing, dizziness, hyperventilation, loose bowels, sweating, muscle tension and insomnia. In some cases, anxiety develops into a panic attack.

Panic attacks are surprisingly common. They are a natural response to anxiety and extreme stress. Many of those who suffer can remember the exact occasion when they experienced their first attack, such as in a crowded super-market or following a series of stressful events at work. If you suffer from panic attacks but cannot remember any particular trigger, some psychologists believe your fear may date from an event in early childhood which is stored in your subconscious memory.

Panic attacks are now thought to be triggered by over-breathing – a condition known as hyperventilation syndrome. During times of extreme stress, your breathing pattern changes as part of the fight or flight response, so you take quick, irregular, shallow breaths that help to draw in more oxygen more quickly. This in turn means you blow off more carbon dioxide – a waste acid gas produced by your metabolism. If you continue hyperventilating, you will soon exhale so much carbon dioxide that your blood loses acidity and becomes increasingly alkaline. This affects the trans-mission of nerve signals and causes physical symptoms of dizziness, faintness and pins and needles. These symptoms heighten your sense of panic, so you tend to breathe even faster, blowing off even more carbon dioxide, and trigger a panic attack. The classic advice to breathe in and out of a paper bag is designed to ensure you re-inhale some of your lost carbon dioxide to replace acidity and relieve your symp-toms.

The most common symptoms experienced during a panic attack are:

- extreme anxiety
- non-specific fears of losing control, embarrassment, rejec-tion or failure
- fluttering in the stomach
- nausea and/or diarrhoea
- rapid pulse

- sweating, especially on the palms
- difficulty breathing or a choking sensation
- pins and needles, especially around the mouth and in the fingers
- blurred vision
- ringing in the ears
- clamminess
- faintness or swooning.

People who habitually hyperventilate sometimes experience frightening physical symptoms, including chest pain, palpitations, visual disturbances, numbness, severe headache, insomnia and even collapse. It is important to seek medical advice if these occur – don't make the diagnosis of panic attack yourself, or it is possible that a more serious problem (e.g. a heart condition) may be missed.

Panic attacks seem to be more common in women than men and researchers have found that middle-aged housewives are the main sufferers, often around the time of the menopause. The reasons are not clear, but it is thought that women who have devoted a major part of their life to being a wife and mother may no longer feel worthwhile once their children leave home, their husband is working long hours and they are home all day on their own. Boredom can lead to feelings of no longer existing as a real, separate individual – something psychiatrists refer to as depersonalization – which can produce extreme anxiety.

Some women find they are more likely to suffer a panic attack just before or during a period. This may be linked with low blood sugar levels, so that symptoms of faintness and light-headedness trigger feelings of anxiety and panic.

To help stop a panic attack:

1. Concentrate on breathing slowly, deeply and quietly to prevent hyperventilation.
2. When you feel panic rising, say 'stop it' quietly to yourself
   - Breathe out deeply, then breathe in slowly to fill your lungs
   - Hold this breath for a count of three then breathe out gently, letting your tension go
   - Continue to breathe regularly and gently; imagine a candle in front of your face – as you breathe, the flame should flicker but not go out
   - While continuing to breathe gently, consciously try to relax so that all your tense muscles unwind.
3. If panic continues to rise, cup your hands over your nose and mouth so you breathe back some of the excess carbon dioxide gas you have blown off.
4. If you are somewhere private, breathe in and out of a paper bag instead.
5. Don't escalate the panic by worrying about what is going to happen.
6. Try to distract your thoughts by studying your surroundings as you wait for the attack to pass – symptoms usually subside quickly.
7. Stay in the situation if practical and you are in no physical danger – if you run away rather than facing your fear, it will be more difficult to cope and to avoid another panic attack when you experience the same situation again.

Relaxation

Relaxation helps to reset the body's stress responses, lowers blood pressure and has a beneficial effect on mind, body and spirit. A number of techniques can help induce relaxation. These include:

- floatation
- massage
- meditation
- qigong
- tai chi chu'uan
- yoga

FLOTATION THERAPY

Flotation therapy involves lying in a light-proof, sound insulated tank containing a shallow pool of saline kept at body temperature. The flotation tank screens out light and sound to remove virtually all external stimulation. This allows the floater to enter a profoundly relaxed state in which they generate theta brainwaves, associated with meditation, creative thought and feelings of serenity. Studies show that you also continue to produce large amounts of theta waves for up to three weeks after a float. You can obtain a similar deep relaxation in your own bath using mineral salts from the Dead Sea (available from larger health food stores and pharmacies).

MASSAGE

Massage forms the basis of many complementary therapies including acupressure, aromatherapy and Shiatsu. Massage is relaxing and can relieve anxiety, tension, aches and pains to sleep as well as lifting a low mood. Combined with relaxing aromatherapy oils the beneficial effects are increased (See Chapter 12).

MEDITATION

Meditation uses the power of the mind to empty itself of thoughts, calm the body and achieve a state of heightened mental or spiritual awareness. By focusing your mind on a particular object or vision, you can screen out distractions and induce a state of profound relaxation and serenity. There are several types of meditation, each of which favour different techniques such as focusing on your breathing rhythm, a universal sound (e.g. Om), a word or phrase with personal meaning (mantra), a physical object (e.g. a flickering candle) or an image. Some techniques involve repetitive movements such as t'ai chi ch'uan or feeling objects such as pebbles or worry beads.

Transcendental Meditation (TM) was developed by Maharishi Mahesh Yogi to be easily practised (15–20 minutes twice a day) despite the busy, modern way of life. TM uses a variety of Sanskrit mantras, each of which is a short word or phrase that, when repeated in the mind, helps the user still their thoughts and find a deeper level of consciousness. This helps you achieve a deep relaxation, while alertness is fully maintained. It leaves you feeling refreshed mentally and physically with a mind that is calmer and able to think more clearly.

QIGONG

Qigong and the related medical therapy, Buqi, are a form of Chinese yoga that combine meditation and posture to achieve relaxation and breath control. Qigong helps to channel energy and calm the mind. The basic postures are easy to learn and – unlike Tai Chi – may be performed in any order.

TAI CHI CHU'UAN

Tai chi chu'uan – also known as Tai Chi – is sometimes

described as meditation in motion. It combines slow, graceful movements with meditation and breathing techniques to calm the mind and improve the flow of the life energy force, Qi. The short form uses 24 slow movements and postures that flow effortlessly one into another and can be performed in five to ten minutes. The long form, consisting of a sequence of 108 movements, takes 20–40 minutes to complete.

YOGA

Yoga combines postural exercises, breathing techniques and meditation to achieve relaxation. A number of yoga forms exist, of which Hatha yoga is most widely practised in the West. Breathing is a major element, as it is viewed as embodying the life force, *prana*, to help achieve emotional and mental harmony.

Sleep

The menopause is often associated with sleeping problems, either due to feelings of anxiety or to the effects of hot flushes and night sweats. This can lead to difficulty in falling asleep, tossing and turning without finding a comfortable position, difficulty staying asleep, having to get up to change the sheets due to excessive sweating and waking up feeling unrefreshed. Recurrent lack of sleep leads to poor performance and achievement during the day. It is also linked with increased risk of serious stress-related illness such as high blood pressure, stroke and even a heart attack.

Sleep is a form of unconsciousness that is our natural state of rest. It is the strongest instinctive urge in humans, yet scientists still do not fully understand how or why we sleep. They do know it is essential for our continued physical and emotional well-being, however. We are designed to spend around a third of our life asleep, yet four out of ten people do not get a regular good night's rest. As a result, they wake up feeling tired, make more mistakes during the day and may repeatedly fall asleep for several seconds at a time. These so-called micro sleeps are a common cause of accidents, both on the roads and in the home.

Sleep patterns seem to change around the time of the menopause, possibly because the brain contains oestrogen receptors, so low levels of oestrogen may have an effect on sleep architecture. After the menopause, women start to spend less and less time in Stage 4 (really deep) sleep, so that by the age of 70, most get no Stage 4 sleep at all. Whereas the average premenopausal women spends around seven hours 12 minutes asleep per night, an older women will naturally often spend as little as five hours asleep.

CAFFEINE, STRESS AND SLEEP

Caffeine – found in tea, coffee, chocolate, soft drinks such as colas as well as some over-the-counter pain killers – is a stimulant drug whose immediate effect is to reduce tiredness and make the body feel alert. Coffee is often consumed in large amounts (e.g. 8–10 cups daily) and as caffeine mimics the effects of adrenaline, causing nervous tension, irritability and insomnia, this can make menopausal symptoms worse as well as interfering with sleep. If you think you are drinking too much coffee, reduce your intake by switching to decaffeinated brands. If stopping caffeine suddenly seems to be making you jittery, gradually reduce your intake by replacing every other cup with a decaffeinated brand then slowly reducing your intake further. Cut back slowly, perhaps by increasing the amount of non-caffeinated coffee you drink, or by switching to tea which contains less caffeine.

To HELP GET A BETTER NIGHT'S SLEEP:

1. Take regular exercise, as active people tend to sleep more easily, but avoid strenuous exercise late in the evening – a gentle stroll round the block is fine.

2. Eat a healthy, low-fat, wholefood diet with plenty of complex carbohydrates (e.g. cereals, bread, pasta) and fruit and vegetables for vitamins and minerals.

3. Try to eat your evening meal before 7.00 p.m. and resist late night snacks, especially of rich food.

4. Avoid over-indulgence in substances that interfere with sleep, such as caffeine nicotine and alcohol – although alcohol may help you fall asleep initially, you are likely to have a disturbed sleep once the drugged effect has worn off.

5. Take time to unwind from the stresses of the day before going to bed – read a book, listen to soothing music or have a candle lit bath.

6. A warm, milky drink just before going to bed will help you to relax – hot milk with cinnamon or nutmeg is better than chocolate drinks that contain some caffeine. Don't drink too much fluid in the evening, however – a full bladder is guaranteed to disturb your rest.

7. Get into a habit by going to bed at a regular time each night and getting up at the same time each morning. Set a bed-time routine such as checking house security, brushing your teeth, bathing and setting the alarm clock to set the mood for sleep.

8. Make sure your bed is comfortable, and your bedroom warm, dark and quiet – noise and excessive cold or heat will keep you awake. A temperature of 18–24 degrees C is ideal.

9. If you can't sleep, don't lie there tossing and turning. Get up and read or watch the television for a while. If you

are worried about something, write down all the things on your mind and promise yourself you will deal with them in the morning, when you are feeling fresher. When you feel sleepy, go back to bed and try again.

10. Preserve your bedroom as a place for sleep (and sex) – don't use it for eating, working or watching television.

NATURAL SLEEP REMEDIES

Sleeping tablets are not a good idea at the best of times and it is also important to avoid over-the-counter sleep medications containing antihistamines. These have been shown in sleep laboratories to give a poor night's sleep with an abnormal sleep architecture, leaving you more drowsy the next day. Fortunately, however, a number of alternative remedies can help diffuse feelings of stress and encourage a natural and restorative sleep.

Supplements containing natural extracts of valerian, lemon balm and hops can induce a refreshing night's sleep without the side-effects associated with drugs.

Soothing herbal teas can also help you sleep. Try infusions of limeflower, lemon balm, fennel, rosehip, passionflower, nutmeg, cinnamon, camomile, valerian or skullcap. It is also worth investing in a herbal pillow filled with dried lavender flowers to place at the head of your bed.

Take the 30 c strength tablet half an hour before going to bed and repeat every 30 minutes if necessary. Use for ten nights then stop and see if your normal sleep pattern has returned.

Aromatherapy can improve sleep problems dramatically (only use under specialist advice during pregnancy). Add 5 drops essential oil to 10 mls (two teaspoons) almond oil and pour into a deep, warm – not hot – bath. Relax in the fragrant water for 15–20 minutes, then sprinkle a few drops

Homeopathy

- If you are wide awake with an over-active mind and can't relax: *Coffea*
- For sleeplessness leaving you irritable and unrefreshed: *Nux vomica*
- If you are overtired physically and mentally and can't get comfortable: *Arnica*
- If kept awake by fear, shock or panic: *Aconitum*
- If you can't sleep and fear you will never do so again: *Ignatia*
- For nightmares that wake you: *Phosphorus*.

of the same essential oil on a cottonwool pad and tuck under your pillow. Choose your favourite fragrance from: camomile, geranium, juniper, lavender, neroli, rose, sandalwood or ylang ylang.

Mix together in blends if you prefer. Vary the oils every four or five days, otherwise you will adapt to it and treatment will be less effective.

The next chapter covers a variety of complementary therapies and treatments, and shows how they can be of benefit during the menopause.

12
Complementary Therapies and the Menopause

Many women with menopausal symptoms find complementary therapies beneficial but, as with orthodox medicine, not every treatment will suit every individual. The skill and training of different therapists also vary widely so, when possible, select a therapist on the basis of personal recommendation from someone whose opinion you trust. Check what qualifications a therapist has and check their standing with the relevant umbrella organisation for that therapy. The organization will be able to tell you what training their members have undertaken, their code of ethics and refer you to qualified practitioners in your area. It is also prudent to find out how long your course of treatment will last and how much it is likely to cost. Don't be afraid to ask how much experience they have had in treating your particular problem(s) and what their success rate is.

Acupuncture

Acupuncture is one of the most ancient and mystical of therapies, having been practised in the Orient for over 4,000 years. Classic acupuncture is based on the belief that we all have a vibrant life energy, known as Qi or Ch'i (pronounced chee) that flows through out-body along special channels known as meridians. The flow of energy through these meridians is believed to depend on the balance of two opposing forces: the Yin and the Yang.

The ancients identified 12 main meridians, six of which have a Yang polarity and are related to hollow organs such as the heart, and six of which have a Yin polarity and are mainly related to solid organs such as the liver. Another eight meridians, which have a controlling function, have also been recognized, making 20 in all.

Qi energy flows along these meridians, and is believed to be concentrated at certain points – known as acupoints – where it can enter or leave the body. Traditionally, 365 acupoints were identified on the meridians, but many more have been now been discovered and around 2,000 acupoints are illustrated on modern charts. Acupoints can now be identified using instruments that measure electrical potentials across the skin. Acupoints have a lower electrical resistance than surrounding areas and can be pinpointed with great accuracy.

In health, energy flows through the meridians in a balanced way. This balance is easily disrupted through factors such as stress, emotions, poor diet and spiritual neglect, however, and in acupuncture, the symptoms of illness are believed to result from imbalances or blockages in energy flow through the body. An acupuncturist will stimulate or suppress the flow of Qi by inserting fine needles into selected acupoints to correct the emotional and physical symptoms of ill health.

Acupuncture can help many menopausal problems, including stress, discomfort, headache, muscle and joint aches and pains, pre-menstrual syndrome, hot flushes, night sweats, as well as emotional problems such as anxiety, depression, insomnia and panic attacks. Most people notice an immediate benefit after just one or two treatments, while with others it may take up to four to six treatments.

Acupuncture is individually tailored to your particular symptoms and signs. Some combinations of points are selected because they are known to help particular problems. Other points may be chosen because they have become tender and painful to touch as a result of abnormal energy flow. These tender points are sometimes known as trigger points or tsubos, and help to indicate where energy imbalance have occurred.

During acupuncture, the therapist inserts a fine, sterile, disposable needle a few millimetres into your skin at each selected acupoint. Many people are put off trying acupuncture because of this use of needles, but it causes surprisingly little, if any, discomfort. You may notice a slight pricking sensation, tingling or buzzing as the needle is inserted or rotated but in the hands of an experienced professional, it really shouldn't hurt at all. Needles are usually left in place for anywhere between ten and 30 minutes and may be occasionally flicked or rotated to stimulate Qi and draw or disperse energy from the point. In some cases, needles may be stimulated with electricity (electroacupuncture) or by burning a small cone of strong-smelling, dried Chinese herb (moxa) – usually wild Mugwort (*Artemisia vulgaris*) near the point to warm the skin. This is known as moxibustion and is believed to stimulate a weak Qi in areas that are cold or painful.

Side-effects are uncommon, as long as you consult a properly trained and experienced practitioner.

Several other complementary treatments are based on the theory that the body's energy flows through channels known as meridians, which lie between the nerves and muscles. These include Acupressure – an ancient oriental technique similar to acupuncture, but instead of inserting needles at points along the meridians to balance the flow of Chi energy, acupoints are stimulated using firm thumb pressure or fingertip massage. Sometimes the therapist will also use their palms, elbows, knees and feet to stimulate different parts of your body. There are three main forms of acupressure massage: Tui Na, Shiatsu and Zero Balancing.

Aromatherapy

Aromatherapy uses aromatic essential oils produced by special glands in the leaves, stems, bark, flowers, roots or seeds of many plants. These oils contain many active ingredients in a highly concentrated and potent form which, because they are volatile, readily evaporate to release their powerful scent. The oils are extracted by a variety of means. Those that are extracted by simple pressing (e.g. bergamot, lemon, orange) are known as essences; those extracted by distillation are known as essential oils; while those obtained by enfleurage (pressing petals between glass sheets coated with animal fat) and solvent extraction are correctly known as absolutes.

Aromatherapy essential oils have powerful effects on mood, as the part of the brain that detects smell messages from the nose is closely linked with the emotional centre in the limbic system. The limbic system is one of the most ancient parts of the brain and is linked to other nerve centres concerned with learning, memories, arousal, emotions and even hormone secretion. Some of these effects are triggered through the production of pheromones – hormone-like substances that have a powerful effect on behaviour even in minute amounts. Oils are also absorbed from the skin into the circulation and can have powerful effects on the body. This is particularly noticeable with some that have diuretic properties.

The sense of smell is more acute in women than men, and menopausal symptoms often respond well to aromatherapy. Several different therapeutic actions may be involved, including:

- the ability to calm, relieve stress and help you relax
- mimicking the effects of natural pheromones or stimulating secretion of your own pheromones
- having an oestrogen-like effect through the plant hormones it contains
- having a testosterone-like effect.

Interestingly, there seem to be no essential oils that have a progesterone-like action. Most have some aphrodisiac properties, too.

Aromatherapy essential oils may be inhaled, massaged into the skin, added to bath water, or heated in a variety of ways to perfume the atmosphere. Where possible, use natural rather than synthetic essential oils. Natural oils generally have a fuller, sweeter aroma that provides a greater therapeutic benefit and. Select 100 per cent pure essential oils – these are usually more expensive, but have a greater effect as they are not mixed with alcohol or other additives.

Dilution

Essential oils that come into contact with skin should always be diluted with a carrier oil (e.g. almond, avocado, jojoba, sunflower, wheatgerm oils). Dilution is important, as oils that are too concentrated may have an adverse effect or cause skin irritation.

Add a maximum total of one drop essential oil to each 2 millilitre (24 drops) of carrier oil. Two teaspoons (10 ml) of carrier oil should therefore contain no more than 5 drops of essential oil blend, while two tablespoons (30 ml) should contain no more than 15 drops of essential oil blend. Oils that are twice as dilute as this often suffice (i.e. only 5 drops essential oil blend per 20 ml carrier oil).

A 5 ml medicinal teaspoon measure (or a 5 ml syringe, if you prefer) can be bought cheaply from a chemist to ensure accuracy, as kitchen teaspoons tend to hold slightly less than 5 ml.

Cautions

- Do not take essential oils internally
- Before using an essential oil blend on your skin, put a small amount on a patch of skin and leave it for at least an hour to make sure you are not sensitive to it
- Do not use essential oils if you are pregnant, or likely to be, except under specialist advice from a qualified aromatherapist
- Do not use essential oils if you suffer from epilepsy, except under specialist advice from a qualified aromatherapist
- Avoid using aromatherapy oils that are known to be capable of putting blood pressure up. These include: thyme, clove and cinnamon
- Keep essential oils away from the eyes
- If you are taking homeopathic remedies, do not use peppermint, rosemary or lavender essential oils, as these may neutralize the homeopathic effect
- Essential oils are flammable, so do not put them on an open flame.

Blends

The best way to use aromatherapy oils is to select two, three or four oils and blend them together to achieve a fragrance you find appealing. Add a maximum total of one drop essential oil to each 2 millilitre (24 drops) of carrier oil.

Oils for Specific Purposes

If you have a particular menopausal problem you are trying to cope with, such as physical exhaustion, low mood, impotence or stress, then include at least one oil in your blend that is useful for helping the problem according to the following table:

	For physical tiredness or mental exhaustion	For low mood or mood swings	For stress or over-work	Relaxing and calming	To help relieve a tension headache	For insomnia
Angelica	•	•				
Clary sage		•	•	•		
Geranium		•	•		•	
Ginger		•				
Grapefruit	•	•	•			
Jasmine		•	•	•		
Juniper berry			•	•		•
Lavender		•	•	•	•	•
Lemon	•	•	•			•
Neroli		•	•	•		•
Orange	•	•	•	•		
Patchouli		•	•			
Pine	•	•				

	For physical tiredness or mental exhaustion	For low mood or mood swings	For stress or over-work	Relaxing and calming	To help relieve a tension headache	For insomnia
Rose		•	•	•	•	•
Rosemary	•				•	•
Sandalwood	•		•	•		•
Vanilla		•	•	•		
Vetiver		•	•	•		
Ylang ylang		•	•	•		•

Oils that are oestrogenic and can help oestrogen withdrawal symptoms include: clary sage, fennel, star anise and tarragon.

Oils that help to relieve hot flushes and sweating include: camomile, clary sage, cypress, geranium, grapefruit, lemon, lime, rose, sage and thyme.

Oils that have diuretic properties include: birch, camomile, cedarwood, fennel, geranium, juniper, lemon and peppermint.

Oils that can help to regulate irregular periods include: basil, camomile roman, clary sage, cypress, fennel, geranium, hyssop, juniper, lavender, marjoram, myrrh, nutmeg, peppermint, rose, rosemary, sage and thyme.

Oils that can help painful periods include: camomile roman, cypress, juniper, nutmeg, peppermint, rosemary, sage and tarragon.

Oils that can help to relieve pre-menstrual symptoms include: anise, bergamot, cardamom, clary sage, cypress, geranium, grapefruit, hyacinth, jasmine, jonquil, lavender, mandarin, rose and sage.

Oils that can help to relieve vaginal dryness include: clary sage, cinnamon, cypress, fennel, geranium, hyacinth, lavender, neroli, nutmeg, melissa, sandalwood and ylang ylang.

Oils that can clear the mind include: basil, grapefruit, rosemary and thyme.

Oils that are antidepressant include: bergamot, camomile, clary sage, geranium, grapefruit, jasmine, lavender, mandarin, melissa, mimosa, neroli, orange, rose, sandalwood and ylang ylang.

Oils with sensual properties that can help to improve low sex drive include: black pepper, jasmine, neroli, patchouli, pimento, rose maroc, rose otto, sandalwood, tuberose, vetiver and ylang ylang.

How to Use Essential Oils

- Make up a relaxing massage oil
- Add to a bath: add 5 drops of essential oils to a tablespoon of carrier oil (e.g. almond, avocado) and mix. Draw your bath so that it is comfortably hot, then add the aromatic oil mix after the taps are turned off. Close the bathroom door to keep in the vapours and soak for 15–20 minutes, preferably in candlelight
- In the shower: add 8 drops of essential oil to a tablespoon (15 ml) of carrier oil. After cleansing your body with soap or gel, rinse well then dip a wet sponge in the oil mix and use it to gently massage your whole body while under a warm jet spray
- To help you sleep: add 2 or 3 drops of a relaxing oil blend to a tissue and allow to dry, before tucking under your pillow
- As a room spray: fill a small sprayer with 100 ml water and add 10 drops of destressing essential oils. Shake the sprayer well before using to perfume your bedroom. This mix can also be placed in special porous holders that will sit over a radiator

- With a ring burner designed to sit over a light bulb so the oils it contains are gently diffused by the heat energy of the bulb
- With a candle-lit diffuser: add 2 or 3 drops of essential oil to a little warm water over a candle burner to diffuse relaxing oils into a room
- With an electric ionizer/diffuser: to fill the room with beneficial negative ions plus a relaxing scent.

Chiropractic

Chiropractic is one of the most popular manipulative therapies, and is widely accepted by the medical profession. Chiropractic is a complementary therapy based on the principle that if joints are poorly aligned or not moving properly, this can affect the function of certain nerves leading to ill health – including more severe menopausal problems.

The nervous system controls every part of the body, through nerves which branch off from the spinal cord and pass through narrow spaces between the bones of the vertebral column. Correct alignment of vertebrae in the spinal column is vital to maintain healthy nerve pathways, and chiropractors specialize in the diagnosis and treatment of conditions that arise from misalignment of these spinal bones. Just a small movement of a vertebra away from its normal position can trap, squash or stretch a nerve and is a common cause of pain, discomfort and reduced mobility. Misalignment of joints can occur for many reasons, including poor posture (e.g. when sitting at a desk, or driving), car accidents, sports injuries, sleeping on a mattress that is overly hard or overly soft, pregnancy and childbirth. Spinal nerve stress can also arise from factors such as poor diet, lack of exercise, anxiety and stress.

The word chiropractic is derived from the Greek *cheir*, meaning *hand*, and *praktikos* meaning *done by*. Chiropractors have a finely tuned sense of touch and use their hands to manipulate and adjust the spine and extremities where there are signs of restricted movement. They typically use rapid, direct, yet gentle thrusts to affected joints in order to realign muscles, tendons, ligaments and bones. The key to the success of these adjustments is in the speed, dexterity and accuracy with which they are performed. This helps to correct poor alignment, improve mobility, relieve pain and tension as well as promoting relaxation. Bones are not forced into place, but adjustments that combine a rapid thrust and immediate release help the bone move towards its correct position. Sometimes, a rubber-tipped instrument known as an Activator is used to gently manipulate the vertebrae, giving a small, precise, measured thrust, especially in older people and infants. Chiropractic may also include stretching and massage techniques if appropriate.

Chiropractors have an holistic approach to health, and manipulation is believed to assist the body's own healing processes, stimulate movement receptors in joints and improve the function of the nervous system. It can help a number of problems that can be associated with the menopause, including headache and pain affecting the muscles or joints.

In 1996, the Royal College of General Practitioners issued guidelines for GPs which recommend manipulative treatment such as chiropractic within the first six weeks for people with low back pain. The report also confirmed that the risks of manipulation are very low in skilled hands. Always tell the practitioner if you have osteoporosis, infection, tumours, inflammatory conditions or circulatory problems, however. While some conditions may not be suitable for full chiropractic treatment, several techniques that provide pain-relief may still be helpful.

During the examination you will be asked to variously stand, sit or lie down on a chiropractic couch and will be manoeuvred into a number of positions to assess your mobility, flexibility and nerve function. This helps the chiropractor assess which joints are moving freely, and which are stiff or locked. This 'motion palpation' assessment is usually accurate enough to identify the exact source of any pain that is troubling you. Irritation of a nerve in one area can sometimes lead to symptoms of discomfort (known as 'referred' pain) in other parts of the body, so manipulation may not be carried out at the site of your pain. For example, tingling in the fingers is often due to misalignment (subluxation) of bones in the neck.

Treatments are generally painless, but you may feel temporary discomfort during an adjustment, that quickly improves. Often, you will have slight aches or stiffness after a session as muscles and joints adapt to their proper alignment.

A chiropractor will often prescribe gentle exercises to help strengthen muscles, and may use ice or heat treatments as appropriate. They will also offer dietary and lifestyle advice, and may suggest nutritional supplements or offer information on other complementary procedures such as magnetic therapy, naturopathy, acupuncture or iridology depending on their special interests. If your problems are related to poor posture, you may also be given ergonomic advice to reduce problems resulting from driving long distances or sitting at a desk for long periods of time.

Homeopathy

Homoeopathy is one of the most popular complementary treatments, as it has a great potential for doing good with little or no risk of causing harm. Homeopathic medicine is based on the belief that natural substances can stimulate the body's own healing powers to relieve the symptoms and signs of illness. The word 'homeopathy' literally means 'similar suffering', and natural substances are selected which, if used full-strength, would produce symptoms in a healthy person similar to those it is designed to treat. In miniscule homeo-pathic doses, however, the opposite effect occurs and symptoms improve. This is the first principle of homoeopathy: *Like Cures Like*.

The second major principle of homeopathy is that increasing dilution of a solution has the opposite effect of increasing its potency, that *Less Cures More*. By diluting noxious substances many millions of times, their healing properties are enhanced, while their undesirable side-effects are lost.

The three Laws of Cure were introduced later. These suggest that when someone is treated with homeopathic remedies: symptoms move from the top of the body down-wards; from the inside out; and from the most important to the least important organs. Symptoms also tend to improve in the reverse order to that in which they appeared.

The way in which homeopathy works is not fully under-stood. It is thought to have a dynamic action that boosts your body's own healing power. The principles that *Like Cures Like*, and *Less Cures More* are difficult concepts to accept, yet convincing clinical trials have shown that homoeopathy is significantly better than inactive substances (placebo) in treating many long-term conditions including hayfever, asthma, migraine, skin problems and rheumatoid arthritis.

The Remedies

Homeopathic remedies are all based on plant, animal or mineral extracts, that are chopped or ground then left to steep in an alcohol/water solution in an airtight jar for two to four weeks, while shaken occasionally. The mixture is then strained off into a dark glass bottle to produce the concentrated mother tincture from which the incredibly diluted homeopathic remedies are made.

Homeopathic remedies are so dilute they are measured on a centesimal scale, in which dilutions of 100^{-6} are described as potencies of 6 c, dilutions of 100^{-30} are written as a potency of 30 c, etc. A 1 c potency dilution is produced by diluting a solution 100 times, by adding 1 drop of the mother tincture (original remedy dissolved in a water/alcohol mix) to 99 drops of a pure water/alcohol solution and shaken and banged (to release the energy of the substance) vigorously. This shaking and banging is known as succussion. To produce a 2 c potency dilution, one drop of the 1 c dilution is added to 99 drops of a pure water/alcohol solution and succussed, and so on. The potency of a homeopathic remedy shows how many times the remedy was diluted like this during its preparation. A remedy with 12 c potency will, therefore, have been diluted by a factor of 100, twelve separate times. To illustrate just how diluted these substances are, a dilution of 12 c (100^{-12}) is comparable to a pinch of salt dissolved in the same volume of water as the Atlantic Ocean. Solutions that are more dilute than 12 c are unlikely to contain even a single molecule of the original substance.

A few drops of a potentized remedy may be added to

lactose (milk sugar) tablets, pillules, powder or granules and swirled together. The lactose tablets, etc. are then stored in an airtight, dark glass bottle, that must be kept out of direct sunlight.

While critics say that homeopathic dilutions contain nothing but water and alcohol, supporters believe the solution is imprinted with the healing energy of the original substance that can stimulate the body's vital force to heal itself. This healing energy may be stored in the way water molecules are aligned, for example, perhaps in a similar way that sounds can be stored on a tape coated in iron filings and later translated back into music when played through a tape recorder.

Constitutional Types

Homeopathic treatments are prescribed according to your symptoms rather than any particular disease, so they are effective for treating a variety of problems. To ensure a person's vital force, or inner healing power, responds as effectively as possible, a practitioner will select the remedy that matches the symptoms and the person as accurately as possible. The homeopath will therefore assess your individual family history, character, lifestyle, likes, dislikes, diet and even the effects of the weather on your symptoms to choose the best remedy for you based on your constitution, i.e. the inherited and acquired physical, emotional and mental factors that make you who you are. A number of constitutional types have been identified, each of which also have a particular remedy that will suit them regardless of the symptoms they are suffering from.

How to Take a Remedy

Although it is best to see a trained homeopath who can assess your constitutional type before deciding which treatment is right for you, remedies can be self-chosen according to your symptoms. Many books and charts are available to help you select an appropriate remedy.

Traditionally, only a single homeopathic remedy is given, for the shortest possible time, to stimulate the body's own healing powers. Some modern remedies contain a number of homeopathic substances however – these are known as combination or complex remedies.

In most cases, you should start with a 6 c potency. Treatment may be taken two or three times a day for up to a week. If partial relief occurs but the symptoms return once you stop taking the remedy, you can increase the effect by taking a 30 c potency.

Homeopathic medicines should ideally be taken on their own, without eating or drinking for at least 30 minutes before or afterwards. Tablets should also be taken without handling – tip them into the lid of the container, or onto a teaspoon to transfer them to your mouth. Then suck or chew them, don't swallow them whole. When taking homeopathic remedies, avoid drinking strong tea or coffee if possible, as these may interfere with the homeopathic effect. Similarly, you should avoid using certain powerful essentials oils such as those of lavender, rosemary and peppermint.

Occasionally, symptoms initially get worse before they get better. This is known as aggravation. Although it is uncommon, try to persevere as it is a good sign that the remedy is working.

Homeopathic Hormones

Homeopathic hormones (oestrogen, progesterone, testosterone and/or oestradiol) are usually prescribed depending on the result of saliva tests. The saliva tests are taken every three days throughout a menstrual cycle, measuring oestrogen, progesterone and testosterone levels. The results are then plotted on a graph to show what hormone changes are occurring during the menstrual cycle, after the menopause or linked with osteoporosis. Homeopathic progesterone may be given in the form of homeopathic Wild Yam cream.

For Period Problems as the Menopause Approaches

Homeopathic remedies that may help irregular periods include:

Pulsatilla 30 c – for women with fair hair and complexion
Sepia 30 c – for brunettes with dark skin
Aconite 30 c – especially if periods stop suddenly due to emotional shock
Ignatia 30 c – especially if periods stop as a result of bereavement
Dose: Take every 12 hours for up to two weeks.

Homeopathic remedies that may help heavy periods include:

Calc carb 30 c – especially if linked with marked premenstrual weight gain
Sepia 30 c – especially if feeling faint, dizzy or irritable
Dose: Take every 8 hours for up to 10 doses.

Homeopathic remedies that may help painful periods include:

Pulsatilla 30 c – especially if feeling weepy
Sepia 30 c – especially if cramping pains are linked with indifference to loved ones
Kali carb 30 c – especially if associated with severe backache
Dose: Take hourly for up to 10 doses.

Homeopathic remedies that may help PMS include:

Sepia 30 c – especially if accompanied by lack of interest
Calc carb 30 c – especially if linked with fluid retention
Pulsatilla 30 c – especially if linked with depression
Dose: Take every 12 hours for up to 6 doses, starting a day before symptoms are expected.

For Physical Menopausal Symptoms

Homeopathic remedies that may help hot flushes include:

Glonoin 30 c – every 5 minutes until flush recedes, for up to 10 doses
Lachesis 30 c – twice a day for up to a week

Homeopathic remedies that may help night sweats include:

Sepia 6 c – for profuse night sweats
Dose: Take hourly for up to 10 doses.

Homeopathic remedies that may help fluid retention include:

Apis 30 c – especially if linked with restlessness and burning hot flushes
Dose: Take every hour for up to 10 doses.

Note: Avoid if you may be pregnant.

Bryonia 6 c – especially if accompanied by painful breasts

Dose: Take every 4 hours for up to 5 days.

Homeopathic remedies that may help vaginal dryness include:

Bryonia 6 c – especially if sore and uncomfortable on movement

Lycopodium 30 c – especially if linked with hot flushes

Dose: Take hourly as necessary, for up to a week.

Homeopathic remedies that may help loss of sex drive include:

Sepia 30 c – especially if loss of interest is severe and linked with exhaustion

Agnus castus 30 c – especially if accompanied by general lowering of energy

Dose: Take every 12 hours for up to a week.

Homeopathic remedies that may help urinary flow problems include:

Sepia 30 c – especially if linked with dragging sensations and difficulty passing water

Causticum 30 c – especially for stress incontinence

Natrum mur 30 c – especially if stress incontinence is linked with vaginal dryness

Dose: Take 4 times a day for up to 3 weeks.

Homeopathic remedies that may help cystitis include:

Cantharis 30 c – especially if you have sudden onset of urinary frequency and burning

Staphysagria 30 c – especially if burning is severe and urine is concentrated

Phosphorus 30 c – especially if burning continues after urination

Dose: Take every 30 minutes for up to 10 doses – seek medical advice if no improvement.

For Emotional menopausal symptoms

Homeopathic remedies that may help anxiety include:

Calc carb 30 c – especially if linked with panic attacks

Lachesis 30 c – especially if talking too much through nervousness

Phosphorus 30 c – especially for constant underlying anxiety

Dose: Take every 12 hours for up to two weeks.

Homeopathic remedies that may help low mood include:

Pulsatilla 30 c: especially if you can't stop crying

Ignatia 30 c – especially if your moods fluctuate wildly

Staphysagria 30 c – especially if sadness is tinged with anger

Nux vomica 30 c – especially if linked with irritability, overwork and stress

Arsen alb 30 c – especially if linked with feelings of restlessness

Dose: Take every 12 hours for up to two weeks.

Homeopathic remedies that may help insomnia include:

Coffea 30 c – especially if you can't relax

Nux vomica 30 c – especially if lack of sleep has made you irritable

Aconite 30 c – especially if sleeplessness is linked with anxiety

Dose: Take 1 hour before going to bed and repeat if you wake up or can't get to sleep.

Homeopathic remedies to help prevent or treat osteoporosis include:

Calc phos – a homeopathic tissue salt used to help bone and teeth problems, including the prevention and treatment of osteoporosis. It is also used to help overcome weakness, exhaustion and fatigue.

Ruta grav – used to help conditions in which the lining of the bone (periosteum) is bruised, with deep aching pain, rheumatism, painful tendons or sciatica. It is sometimes used to help treat osteoporosis where the bone has been damaged.

Theridion – mainly acts on the nerves, spine and bones and is useful for helping people with spinal osteoporosis.

Bryonia – used to treat painful conditions that come on slowly, including influenza, headaches, osteoarthritis, rheumatism and other bone problems, including osteoporosis.

After completing a course of homeopathy, you will usually feel much better in yourself with a greatly improved sense of well-being that lets you cope with any remaining symptoms in a much more positive way.

Homeopathic Bach Flower Remedies

Bach Flower Remedies are homeopathic preparations in which flower essences are preserved in grape alcohol (brandy). They are unusual remedies in that they do not treat physical symptoms, but instead rebalance emotions and treat negative mental states such as worry, anxiety, despondency and guilt. They are especially helpful for the variety of emotional states that may be associated with the menopause.

Flower remedies were devised earlier this century when a homoeopathic doctor, Edward Bach, realized that people suffering from the same emotional problems benefited from the same homeopathic treatment, irrespective of the physical symptoms they were suffering. This led him to the belief that physical symptoms were due to underlying emotional stresses which, if not remedied, would inevitably lead to more serious future illness. He classified emotional problems into seven major groups, which he then subdivided into a total of 38 negative or harmful states of mind. For each of these emotional states, he then identified a complementary flower essence that could restore emotional balance.

Bach flower remedies are prepared either by infusion or boiling. In the infusion method, flower heads are placed on the surface of a small glass bowl filled with pure spring water. This is left to infuse in direct sunlight for three hours, then the flowers are discarded and the infused spring water preserved in grape alcohol (brandy). This resultant solution is called the mother tincture, which is further diluted to create the individual stock remedies.

In the boiling method, short lengths of twig-bearing flowers or catkins are boiled in pure spring water for 30 minutes. The plant material is then discarded and the water allowed to cool before being preserved in grape alcohol. The resultant solution is the mother tincture which will be further diluted for use.

The remedies are available over-the-counter in chemists and health food shops. Although the easiest way to take them is to put two drops from the bottle onto your tongue, this does use up a lot of remedy, and is less convenient if you are taking more than one remedy at a time. It is usually better to take the remedies in water. To do this, put two drops of each selected remedy into a glass of water and sip from the glass until the feelings have passed. You can mix together up to seven remedies at a time.

A useful option is to make up a treatment bottle using an empty 30 ml dropper bottle. Add two drops of each selected remedy and top up with non-fizzy mineral water. If you wish, you can also add a teaspoon of brandy to help the water stay fresh. You then take four drops of this treatment remedy four times a day – although it can be used more frequently if you need it.

RESCUE REMEDY

The most famous Bach Flower Remedy is Rescue Remedy – a pre-mixed combination of Rock Rose, Impatiens, Clematis, Star of Bethlehem and Cherry Plum for use in times of crisis or life's ups and downs. Rescue Remedy helps to counteract faintness, shock and loss of self-control. Add four drops of Rescue Remedy to a glass of water and sip slowly, every three to five minutes, holding the liquid in your mouth for a while. Alternatively, place four drops directly under your tongue. It is useful for any acute recurrences of symptoms that leave you feeling unable to cope, such as when a hot flush, night sweat or panic attack strikes.

Bach Flower Remedies useful during the menopause include:

FOR FEAR

Aspen (*Populus tremula*) – for vague fears and anxieties of unknown origin, sense of foreboding, apprehension or impending doom

Cerato (*Ceratostigma willmottianum*) – for those who doubt their own ability to judge situations or make decisions

Scleranthus (*Scleranthus annus*) – for the indecisive and those subject to energy or mood swings

Hornbeam (*Carpinus betulus*) – for 'Monday morning' feelings of not being able to face the day, tiredness, procrastination and those needing inner strength

Olive (*Olea europaea*) – for total exhaustion, mental or physical; weariness, sapped vitality, especially during convalescence

White Chestnut (*Aesculus hippocastanum*) – for persistent, unwanted thoughts, mental arguments, preoccupation with worry

Mustard (*Sinapis arvensis*) – for deep gloom descending for no apparent reason, melancholy and heavy sadness

Walnut (*Juglans regia*) – for stabilizing the emotions during periods of transition, (e.g. puberty, menopause); – for adjusting to new beginnings or relationships

Elm (*Ulmus procera*) – for those who overextend themselves, are overwhelmed or burdened with responsibilities

Oak (*Quercus robur*) – for the brave and determined, who never usually give up despite adversity or illness, but who are losing their strength to fight

Chicory (*Cichorium intybus*) – for those who like to keep their family and friends close by, and find it difficult to allow them to go their own way; for people who expect dutiful obedience in return for the love they give.

Magnetic Therapy

Like acupuncture, Magnetic therapy can also be used to access the body's electric and magnetic fields by stimulating acupoints with tiny pulses of electromagnetic energy. This is most easily achieved using rare earth magnets made from an alloy of neodymium, iron and boron (known as Acumed). These are coated with purified zinc and surrounded with tiny copper spheres, which generate an electric field when connected by sweat on the skin surface. These therapeutic electromagnets are pre-attached to adhesive patches and can be stuck to the skin over particular acupuncture points – or areas of tenderness (tsubos) – to relieve pain and stiffness associated with conditions as diverse as arthritis, rheumatic condition, headache, menstrual pain, insomnia and lack of energy. Patches are left undisturbed for five to seven days.

Magnetic therapy acts on nerve and muscle cells to relieve pain, relax tense muscles, improve the circulation, boost immunity and energy levels.

Osteopathy

Osteopathy is now widely accepted by the medical profession. It is a method of diagnosis and treatment based on the mechanical structure of the body's musculo-skeletal system. Osteopaths believe that the muscles, ligaments, connective tissues, bones and joints don't just form a coat-hanger to support your body, but are also important in maintaining the health of other parts of the body such as the respiratory and digestive systems. Gentle manipulation of the soft tissues and joints is used to help relax muscles, correct poor alignment, improve body function, reduce pain and restore health.

Osteopathy can also help other problems not obviously related to the joints and muscles, as misalignment of the joints is believed to disrupt nerve supply to other vital organs so they function less efficiently. It is therefore used to improve some menopausal symptoms such as headache, dizziness, menstrual pain, insomnia and depression.

An osteopath uses their sense of touch to palpate (feel) parts of the body to detect any areas of weakness or excessive strain. Your posture will be checked for symmetry and alignment of the pelvis and the length of your legs is compared. Manipulation is not usually painful, but this will depend on the underlying problem – if you feel uncomfortable, don't be afraid to say so. Often, blood pressure is measured and nerve reflexes tested by gently tapping on muscle tendons at the knee, ankle, elbows and/or wrists using a small rubber reflex hammer.

Osteopaths use their hands to perform a wide range of manipulations on the body. These can include gentle massage, soft tissue techniques to relax tension, rhythmic passive joint mobilizations to improve the range of movement in a joint, and swift, high velocity thrusts that can produce impressive cracking sounds. Gentle release techniques are most widely used.

Cranial Osteopathy

Cranial osteopathy is a modern extension to osteopathy developed in the 1930s, when it was found that the fused bones making up the dome of the skull retain slight flexibility. Altogether, there are 26 bones in the head. At birth, the bones making up the dome of the skull are not joined, and can overlap one another to make childbirth easier. By age 13, the bones have formed some joints, known as sutures, but these are not fully developed until after the age of 18. For some reason, the bones do not fuse to form a solid block, but can flex slightly so the head becomes slightly wider from side to side, and slightly shorter from front to back, when breathing in.

Cranial osteopaths believe this happens to accommodate natural movements within the cerebrospinal fluid (CSF) that bathes and nourishes the brain and spinal cord, which is said to pulsate at six to 15 times per minute. Practitioners sense this pulsation (known as the cranial rhythmic impulse) with their hands and 'listen' to the inner movements and tensions inside the patient. An osteopath then uses their highly trained sense of touch to identify and correct disturbances in the joints of the skull, which are then manipulated using gentle but specific adjustments to improve circulation of CSF, blood and lymph in the head. The technique is gentle enough to use even on tiny babies.

Cranial osteopathy can help a wide range of conditions, including menopausal problems and stress associated with them.

Craniosacral Therapy

Craniosacral therapy is a version of cranial osteopathy developed in the 1970s, and involves gentle manipulation of both the skull and base of the spine. Practitioners believe that the cranial rhythmic impulses affect every cell in the body due to the continuity of fluids and tissues within the skull and spinal column, so that the head (cranium) and a bone in the back of the pelvis (sacrum) work together as a single unit. Gently manipulating and pressing on the head and sacrum aims to ensure an even, rhythmic flow of the cranial rhythmic impulse, to release inner tensions over a wide area. Many osteopaths practise these techniques with great success, and most people experiencing craniosacral therapy feel deeply relaxed during the treatment, and notice spontaneous unwinding of tension due to the release of physical and emotional imbalances.

Craniosacral therapy can help the same range of conditions as standard osteopathy, including back and neck pain, headache, insomnia, stress, anxiety and digestive disorders.

13
Hormone Replacement and Other Drug Therapies

While diet and lifestyle changes and herbal remedies are important to help reduce the short- medium- and long-term effects of oestrogen withdrawal after the menopause, there are times when prescribed treatments may be desirable. Medications are available that can ease short-term menopausal symptoms such as hot flushes, night sweats and mood swings; help to minimize the development of menopausal symptoms such as vaginal dryness and stress incontinence, and which may postpone or minimize your risk of long-term post-menopausal problems such as osteoporosis.

These drug therapies include:

- *Clonidine* – a non-hormone drug that prevents blood vessel dilation and may help to improve hot flushes and night sweats if you are unable to take HRT
- *Hormone Replacement Therapy (HRT)*

- *Selective Estrogen Receptor Mediators (SERMs)* which have beneficial protective effects against osteoporosis
- *Natural Progesterone*
- *Biphosphonate tablets* (e.g. alendronic acid, etidronate) that help to protect against osteoporosis by slowing the rate of bone turn over and stimulating production of new bone
- *Calcitonin* – a hormone injection derived from salmon, which helps to regulate bone turn over and increases bone density in women with osteoporosis.

These are discussed in greater detail below.

Clonidine

HRT is not the only drug option to treat distressing menopausal symptoms. Clonidine is sometimes prescribed to reduce hot flushes, as it helps to prevent dilation of blood vessels. Clonidine is taken morning and evening and usually controls flushing and night sweats quite well. Its use is limited by side-effects however, that can include drowsiness, dry mouth, dizziness, nausea, constipation, sleeplessness and occasional rashes, although most women tolerate it well.

Hormone Replacement Therapy (HRT)

Two and a half million women now use some form of hormone replacement therapy, for which six million prescriptions, costing an estimated £150 million, were issued in England alone during 2001.

Hormone replacement therapy was introduced into the UK in 1956, when it was hailed as one of the most exciting and beneficial developments in maintining optimum health for older women. Sadly, its promise does not seem to have matched by the clinical experience, and the balance of risks and benefits for hormone use in healthy, post-menopausal women remains uncertain. Its main use remains in alleviating short-term symptoms of hot flushes and night sweats. Long-term trials suggest it does not offer the expected benefits against long-term risk of coronary heart disease, although it does seem to protect against osteoporosis if taken for long enough. Against this, however, is its association with a small increased risk of breast cancer, which is the main reason why HRT is not usually prescribed for more than ten years after a woman has reached the age of 50.

HRT has always been controversial, but recently it has come under renewed attack. Research findings that oestrogen therapy was linked with an increased risk of ovarian cancer were closely followed by news that a large clinical trial in the US had been abandoned after five years due to an unexpectedly high increased risk of heart disease, stroke and breast cancer.

The HRT and Ovarian Cancer Trial

Research published in the *Journal of the American Medical Association* (JAMA) found that women who had used oestrogen-only HRT for 20 years were almost three times more likely to develop ovarian cancer than those not taking it. Although these relative figures seem high, the absolute, individual risk for each woman still remains low. Out of 100,000 women who have never used HRT, around 26 would be expected to die from ovarian cancer. What this study found was that for women using oestrogen-only HRT for ten or more years, the figure was increased to 64 women per 100,000. This study found no significant link between ovarian cancer and using combined oestrogen-progestogen HRT. There also appeared to be minimal risk associated with short-term use, although further research is needed. For women who have had a hysterectomy while retaining their ovaries, it now seems that long-term use of oestrogen-only HRT is unwise.

The Abandoned Trial

Around 16,000 women, aged 50 to 79, who had not had a hysterectomy, took part in the American Women's Health Initiative study which was planned to run for eight years. Half received an oestrogen-progestogen combined HRT tablet providing 0.625 mg conjugated equine oestrogens plus 2.5mg medroxyprogesterone acetate daily, while the other half received inactive placebo. After five years, however, participants were advised to stop taking the HRT combination, three years earlier than planned, as accumulating data suggested that, for this particular blend of HRT, the benefits did not outweigh the risks. This form of HRT was found to increase the risk of breast cancer by 26 per cent, the risk of coronary heart disease by 29 per cent and the risk of a stroke by 41 per cent, with a lack of overall benefit.

If you are taking HRT, it is important not to panic as, although these figures seem high, the overall risk for each individual woman remained low and, importantly, the risk of dying was not increased as a result of therapy. The researchers estimated that for every 10,000 women taking HRT, it would have accounted for an extra eight cases of invasive breast cancer, eight more strokes, eight additional blood clots affecting the lung and seven heart attacks per year. The particular HRT product involved in this trial is not available in the UK, and these side-effects may not be applicable to other HRT formulations.

In 2002, it was also revealed at the annual conference of the British Society for Gastroenterology that women who take HRT for two or more years are over three times more likely to develop gallstones than women who do not use HRT. In the same year, researchers in Oxford found that taking HRT triples the risk of a potentially fatal blood clot from one in 10,000 to three in 10,000.

HRT is therefore fast falling from favour. News that lawyers in America have now launched a worldwide class action on behalf of women who believe HRT has harmed them has added even more fuel to the flames. So where does this leave women who are currently taking hormone replacement therapy?

There are some positives attached to it. There is no doubt that HRT is effective in relieving hot flushes, night sweats, vaginal dryness and some urinary symptoms. It can also reduce the risk of a hip fracture by 30 per cent and the risk of a spinal fracture by as much as 50 per cent. It must be taken for a minimum of seven to ten years to achieve this optimum level of bone protection, however. Researchers have also found that taking HRT seems to reduce the risk of bowel cancer. Out of 12 studies involving over 5,000 people with cancer of the bowel, five found a 20 per cent to 40 per cent reduction in risk for women who had previously used HRT, with the protective effect being strongest in recent users. Further studies are needed to confirm this finding. Other long-term benefits of HRT that are less well known include improved dental health, with less receding of gums and loss of teeth related to the beneficial effects of oestrogen on bone in the jaw.

Most women start HRT to treat menopausal symptoms such as hot flushes, night sweats and vaginal dryness, and only use it short term until their symptoms have subsided. On average, British women only take HRT for nine months. Short-term use of HRT for less than five years appears to be associated with only a small increased risk of serious side-effects. The benefits are usually thought to outweigh the risks, as it can greatly improve quality of life at what can be a very difficult time. However, every woman is different, and her individual needs, personal and family history will play a role in whether or not she chooses to take HRT, and whether her GP is prepared to prescribe it. Decisions about taking HRT involve very personal, subjective judgements. Some women regard the small increased risk of breast cancer as more important than the reduction in risk of heart disease – especially if a friend or relative has suffered. Other women may prefer to prevent an immobilizing hip fracture or painful osteoporotic collapse of their vertebrae resulting in disfiguring spinal deformities.

Where HRT is indicated, it is usually prescribed for as long as is needed to take you up until the age of 50. After this age it can then be prescribed for a further ten years. Few doctors would not prescribe it for more than ten years over the age of 50, as this would increase the possible risk of breast cancer beyond that which is currently felt acceptable.

Only you can decide whether you feel comfortable taking hormone replacement therapy, and for how long. The important thing is to have all the information at your fingertips so you can make an informed choice. This means questioning your doctor about the possible benefits and risks of HRT to you, bearing in mind your past medical history, lifestyle, inheritable family illnesses such as osteoporosis, heart disease or breast cancer, plus the effects of any other medications you are taking.

If you have been, or were planning, to take HRT long term, you should talk to your doctor about the risks involved and whether you should continue. It may be that other treatment is now considered more suitable. And where HRT is no longer recommended, it is even more important to take diet and lifestyle measures to reduce your risk of heart disease and stroke. These include maintaining a healthy weight, eating a healthy diet, taking regular exercise and taking calcium and vitamin D supplements to strengthen your bones.

Doctors' Attitudes to the Menopause and HRT

Different doctors have different attitudes to the menopause and HRT. Some doctors feel very positive about HRT, while others are against it for various reasons. Interestingly, female doctors are twice as likely to take HRT themselves than women who are not involved in healthcare, and most take it for more than five years.

If your doctor has a set opinion about the menopause and HRT, it can sometimes be difficult to obtain the information you need, and to receive full counselling about which treatment option is right for you. Don't be afraid to ask your doctor, practice nurse or pharmacist for more information. Some useful addresses where you can obtain extra advice are also available at the end of this book.

If you feel your doctor is not as sympathetic to your problems as you would like, or if you feel rushed or undecided, you can ask to be referred to a gynaecologist or to a special menopause clinic. There are usually available in larger NHS hospitals.

If you are unable, or unwilling, to take HRT,

non-hormonal methods of helping to relieve menopausal symptoms are also available (see Chapters 8 and 12).

A number of fact sheets, including one entitled *HRT – its Pross and Cons*, are available from the Natural Menopause Advice Service (see Useful Addresses for contact details).

What is Hormone Replacement Therapy?

Hormone replacement therapy is a way of giving you back the oestrogen hormone that your ovaries can no longer produce in large amounts. HRT aims to restore hormonal equilibrium by returning your oestrogen levels to their normal, pre-menopausal state. In fact, HRT is designed to give you back average levels of oestrogen so that – over the course of a month – you receive the same, or less, oestrogen than if your ovaries were continuing to work at their normal, pre-menopausal rate.

HRT may be prescribed for a number of reasons, including:

- To prevent a premature menopause in women whose ovaries are removed
- The relief of menopausal symptoms such as hot flushes, night sweats and mood swings
- To treat vaginal dryness or stress incontinence
- To reduce your lifetime risk of osteoporosis.

The only hormone replacement believed to be needed is oestrogen – the other female hormone, progesterone, is thought by most researchers to be less important from a health and symptom point of view. Some doctors feel the opposite is true, however, and that progesterone may be more important than oestrogen although this is controversial.

Oestrogen can only be given on its own if you have had a hysterectomy, however. It cannot be given alone if you still have an intact uterus, as this would produce over-stimulation of the womb lining (endometrium) causing it to plump up excessively. Over a period of time, this might result in abnormal cell changes (cystic hyperplasia) that have been linked with an increased risk of endometrial cancer. A synthetic form of progesterone is therefore given as well, during the last ten to 14 days of each menstrual cycle. This protects your womb lining from over-stimulation and is known as combined HRT. Combined HRT mimics a normal menstrual cycle and produces a regular bleed similar to a light period. This bleeding is not really a period, however, and is more correctly known as a withdrawal bleed.

If you have previously had a hysterectomy though, this problem does not arise. You can be prescribed oestrogen-only HRT without having to take cyclical progesterone.

THE HORMONES USED IN HRT

There are at least 50 different brands of HRT, which in turn are often available in different doses. This range of choice is important, as it allows a doctor to select a blend of hormones that will suit each individual woman.

Different blends of HRT contain different types of oestrogen hormone. Often, a natural form of oestrogen is used that is identical to the oestrogens in your own body (oestradiol, oestrone and oestriol). A synthetic oestrogen that is slightly different from natural oestrogen is also occasionally used (ethinyloestradiol). Oestrogens that are described as 'conjugated' are in a form that is closely similar to those occurring in your body.

Natural progesterone itself cannot be taken by mouth, as it is quickly broken down in the stomach. Synthetic forms – known as a progestogen – are therefore used, of which several different ones are available (e.g. dydrogesterone, levonorgestrel, medroxyprogesterone, norethisterone, norgestrel).

One synthetic hormone (tibolone) has both oestrogen-like and progestogen-like actions. This means that it can be given on its own, without the need for a separate progestogen, even in women who have not had a hysterectomy. It is only prescribed for post-menopausal women who have not had a natural menstrual period for at least a year, however.

When you start taking HRT, your doctor has to select the blend he or she thinks will suit you best. If a particular blend of HRT does not seem to suit you, switching to another formulation containing a different oestrogen or progestogen, or changing the dose you are taking, will often solve the problem. While many women are quite happy with the first brand of HRT they take, some try two, three or even more doses or blends of hormones as their doctor tailors HRT to their individual situation. Try not to be put off if this happens to you. One of the advantages of having such a variety of HRT available is that most women eligible to take HRT eventually find one that suits.

HRT and Menstruation

Early forms of HRT, in which cyclical progesterone was given to prevent over-stimulation of the endometrium, meant the return of a regular monthly bleed for women who had not had a hysterectomy. Not surprisingly, this put a lot of women off taking HRT. This monthly bleed is not a period as such, but a withdrawal bleed due to the changing levels of progesterone present in the formulation to protect your womb lining as described above. With newer formulations, however, advances mean that if you have not had a period for at least a year, taking HRT no longer has to mean the inevitable return of a monthly bleed – you may only have to have one every three months, or not at all.

Continuous V Cyclical HRT

Women who have not had a hysterectomy need to take combined oestrogen and progestogen HRT. The progestogen can be given in two ways:

1. In cycles that last one month or three months
2. Continuously, in which the oestrogen and progestogen are given together, every day, without interruption.

The most suitable regime depends on your menopausal status: if you are still having a natural menstrual bleed, or are within one year of your last natural menstrual period, you will need cyclical HRT; if you are post-menopausal *and* over 54 years of age, or if you had your last natural menstrual period more than one year previously, you can receive continuous combined HRT.

The difference between the these methods is an important one for most women. When the progestogen is given in cycles, you will still have a light, withdrawal bleed. If the progestogen cycle is one month long, you will have a bleed every four weeks. If the progestogen cycle is three months long, you will only bleed once every quarter.

If you are eligible for continuous, combined hormone replacement therapy, treatment usually remains period-free. You may still experience light bleeding or spotting during the first few months of use while your body adapts to the new hormone regime. Because you are receiving the progestogen continuously, your womb lining is still protected against over-stimulation and your risk of womb cancer is still reduced.

If you currently use a form of cyclical HRT that means you have a period every month and you would prefer to have a period only every three months, this is something you should discuss with your doctor. Your pharmacist can also give you further information. If you are using a cyclical form of HRT with regular bleeds, you may be able to take a continuous combined form of HRT that is usually period-free. This will only be the case if you: have received treatment for one to two years; *or* had stopped having periods for a time before starting HRT; *or* are over 54 years of age.

Endometrial Cancer

After five years of using oestrogen-only HRT in women who have not had a hysterectomy, the risk of endometrial cancer is increased more than six-fold and this is not recommended. In the US, however, some doctors prescribe oestrogen alone to women who have not had a hysterectomy and monitor the womb lining for changes through regular biopsies. The relative risk of endometrial cancer is reduced to three times normal with 10 days added progestogen, to less than twice normal risk with cyclical progestogen, and further reduced to 0.2 (ie 80 per cent below normal risk for non users) when oestrogen is opposed with continuous progestogens. Continuous progestogen therapy may therefore be the way forward when prescribing long-term oestrogen replacement therapy, especially in those continuing treatment beyond the age of 60 years.

Different Formulations Available

New ways of taking HRT are becoming available all the time – the range has never been greater, which means that most women are able to find a formulation that suits them, assuming they are happy to take it and are eligible for therapy. Preparations that are currently available include:

- oral tablets
- skin patches
- skin gels
- implants
- vaginal creams
- vaginal pessaries
- vaginal tablets
- a nasal spray.

An intra-uterine progestogen coil used together with oral oestrogen tablets is available in some countries.

If you are not happy with the type of HRT you are using – for example, because you forget to take a tablet, find the vaginal cream messy, or you would prefer to try a patch or gel, don't be afraid to discuss this with your doctor.

When HRT is taken by mouth, a larger dose is usually needed than when hormones are absorbed through your skin (e.g. implants, patches, gels, creams, nasal spray). This is because hormones absorbed from your stomach travel to your liver, where they are partially broken down before they reach their final destinations. HRT tablets are therefore more likely to cause minor side-effects. If you are having problems finding an HRT tablet to suit you, ask your doctor whether another formulation such as a patch or gel would suit you best.

Oral Tablets

If you have had a hysterectomy and are taking oestrogen-only HRT, you will need to take a tablet regularly, every day, without a pill-free break.

If you are taking a combined oestrogen and progestogen preparation, you will usually be prescribed a pack contain a course of 21, 28 or 91 daily tablets:

- tablets containing oestrogen are taken regularly throughout the cycle
- the tablets containing the progestogen are taken during the last ten to 14 days of the cycle. These will either be a separate tablet, taken together with the oestrogen treatment, or a combined tablet containing both hormones.

Some formulations mean you have a seven-day, tablet-free break in which you will experience a light withdrawal bleed resembling a period.

Most formulations mean you take a tablet regularly, every day, starting one 28-day course after another. The tablets contain different blends of oestrogen and progestogen so that your period comes regularly, once a month, while you are still taking the tablets. With the newer three-monthly type of HRT, you take a tablet continuously for 91 days (one colour tablet for 70 days, a second colour for 14 days and a third colour for seven days), but only have a withdrawal bleed once every three months.

Skin Patches

HRT skin patches contain hormones that slowly pass from the patch into the skin. An HRT patch is stuck on to the skin of your bottom, lower abdomen or hips and changed regularly every three to four days (twice a week).

A patch can be used for:

- continuous oestrogen-only HRT
- cyclical combined HRT (with the progestogen either included in the patch for part of the month, or given separately by mouth)
- continuous combined period-free HRT (oestrogen and progestogen given together without a break for those who are eligible – see above).

Each patch should be removed and discarded when a new one is used. Skin patches can occasionally fall off and may release excess hormone in hot weather, or during vigorous exercise. Around one in 20 women using a skin patch develops slight skin irritation, although this is rarely troublesome. Simple measures such as avoiding using talcum powder or body lotion before applying the patch will help the patch stick to your skin more easily. A new patch should be applied to a different area of skin from the one it is replacing, to minimize local skin reactions such as redness or itching. If irritation occurs, it is often due to a small amount of alcohol contained in the adhesive. If this happens, try removing the backing from a patch and then wait ten minutes before applying the patch to your skin. This lets the alcohol evaporate and reduces the chance of irritation.

Skin Gels

Oestrogen-only HRT can be given as a clear, colourless gel that is dispensed from a canister (or individual sachets) and rubbed into the skin of your arm, shoulder or inner thigh.

Two measures are used once a day – increased to four measures after a month if necessary. Oestrogen gel may be used together with progestogen tablets in women where an opposed HRT regime is needed.

Implants

An oestrogen implant is a small hormone store that is inserted under the skin of your lower abdomen. It is usually only prescribed for women who have had a hysterectomy. It can be implanted during your hysterectomy operation, or in your GP surgery using local anaesthetic to numb the skin. Once an oestrogen implant is in place, it slowly releases a steady amount of hormone into your circulation over the following four to eight months before dissolving and disappearing.

Vaginal Cream, Pessaries and Tablets

If your menopausal symptoms mainly consist of urinary or vaginal problems (e.g. leakage, dryness or discomfort), you and your doctor may decide that you only need local oestrogen replacement treatment with a cream, pessary or vaginal tablet. This will reduce vaginal dryness, reverse tissue shrinkage and increase lubrication.

Oestrogen creams are inserted into the vagina using a special applicator which you fill with cream yourself. At first, you use the cream once or twice a day, then you can drop down to using it one to three times a week. Every few months, your doctor will re-examine you and the dose may be reduced or discontinued, depending on how well your tissues have responded to treatment.

Oestrogen can also be delivered locally to the vagina in the form of a pessary or a vaginal tablet. The two are very similar, although a pessary tends to be larger and made of a softer material that quickly melts at body temperature. Oestrogen pessaries are used by inserting two pessaries at night for two to three weeks only.

Oestrogen vaginal tablets are inserted with a special applicator – one tablet daily for two weeks, reduced to one tablet twice a week for ten weeks. Treatment is then usually discontinued to assess your need for further treatment, and repeated as necessary.

Oestrogen delivered into the vagina is usually low dose and is not greatly absorbed into your bloodstream. This means it does not usually help hot flushes or sweats, and does not normally over-stimulate the womb lining. These treatments need getting used to as they can be messy, however. They are useful for short-term treatment of vaginal or urinary problems though. If you decide to use them long term, and have not had a hysterectomy, you may need to take a cyclical progestogen for ten to 14 days each month with some preparations. Your doctor, practice nurse or pharmacist can give you more information.

Note: Many HRT cream formulations damage the latex of rubber condoms and diaphragms.

Nasal Spray

Oestrogen nasal spray is used initially once daily into each nostril at around the same time of day. The dose can be increased to up to four sprays daily in divided doses. It can be used every day or for just 21 to 28 days followed by a two to seven day treatment free interval. Women with a uterus must also receive a progestogen (e.g. tablet) for at least 12 days of each cycle. If you have a severely blocked nose, the spray can be given into the mouth between the cheek and gum temporarily, in which case the normal dose should be doubled.

When Should I Start Taking HRT?

Your oestrogen levels will start to fall during the five years before your last period ends. During this time, you may experience hot flushes, sweats and vaginal dryness.

HRT can be started before your periods stop if your menopausal symptoms are troublesome, especially if your periods have become infrequent. This will usually greatly relieve your menopausal symptoms within seven to ten days.

If you have had a hysterectomy with removal of your ovaries, you will usually be started on HRT – either immediately (e.g. if an oestrogen implant is inserted into your scar during the operation), or shortly afterwards.

There is no upper age limit for starting HRT. Some women in their nineties have started it, for example, to help treat osteoporosis, or urinary leakage due to tissue shrinkage. Most women start HRT around the time of their menopause, or soon after, however. After the age of 50, HRT should not usually be taken for more than ten years to reduce any possible increased risk of breast cancer.

What are the Immediate Benefits?

Taking oestrogen replacement therapy quickly improves the short-term symptoms of oestrogen withdrawal. Some women opt to take HRT for only six to 12 months until the worst of their menopausal symptoms are over. If HRT suits you, however, you will gain long-term benefits that help to protect you against osteoporosis, if you can continue taking it for as long as recommended.

What are the Long-term Benefits of HRT?

There is good evidence that taking small doses of HRT for several years, starting around the time of the menopause, will help to reduce your risk of osteoporosis and may also reduce memory loss. For women who have not had a hysterectomy, taking combined HRT (oestrogen plus a progestogen) also seems to reduce the risk of cancer of the womb lining (endometrium). To obtain the long-term benefits of HRT against osteoporosis, it must be taken for at least seven years. For women who have had a hysterectomy and experienced a premature menopause, HRT should be taken up until the age of 50 (when they would otherwise have reached the menopause), before the clock starts ticking and these additional seven years start being counted.

HRT and Osteoporosis

Oestrogen is important for stimulating production of new bone to replace old bone that has been recycled. Once oestrogen levels fall after the menopause, less new bone is made, so as old bone is recycled, the risk of osteoporosis increases (see Chapter 7). Oestrogen replacement slows bone loss and also improves the quality of new bone produced, so that it is stronger and less likely to fracture. Overall, it seems that HRT can reduce the risk of a hip fracture by up to 30 per cent and spinal fracture by 50 per cent. Oestrogen replacement has been shown to prevent bone loss when treatment starts up to six years beyond the time of the menopause, but needs to be continued for at least seven years for optimum benefits. Several studies have also looked at the benefits of starting HRT in women aged over 60, of which three randomized, controlled trials, showed an increase in bone mass of 4.7 per cent to 9.9 per cent.

Although bone loss continues once oestrogen therapy stops, HRT buys your bones extra thickness, so they are less likely to become brittle during your natural life span. Some doctors are concerned about using HRT long term for more than seven years, and prefer to have a discussion with the woman concerned at this stage so that she can make the final decision about whether or not to stay on HRT. This is because the cardiovascular benefits of long-term HRT seem to be less certain, and because alternative treatments to protect against osteoporosis (e.g. raloxifene) are now available.

HRT and Heart Disease

After the menopause, a woman's risk of a heart attack rapidly increases until it is two or three times that of pre-menopausal women of the same age. Early trials seemed to suggest that taking oestrogen replacement therapy could halve the risk of a heart attack in some women. The issue is much less clear-cut than previously thought, however, with one recent large trial seeming to suggest that at least one blend might even increase the risk of coronary heart disease. Some doctors still feel that oestrogen replacement therapy remains an important strategy in preventing CHD in some post-menopausal women – most likely due to its beneficial effects on blood fat levels. It is important to have the full pros and cons explained to you before taking HRT for this reason, however.

Alzheimer's Disease

Alzheimer's disease is a form of senile dementia (see page 87). Women are affected more than men and some research has suggested that oestrogen HRT can help to reduce the risk of developing Alzheimer's disease by around one third.

Why do Women Stop Using HRT?

Around one in three women stop taking HRT within six months, with half discontinuing within 12 months.

A woman may decide to stop taking HRT for a number of reasons – many because their menopausal symptoms of hot flushes have resolved on treatment and they feel they no longer need it, perhaps the ideal situation in those with no increased risk of osteoporosis. Around one in four women stop taking HRT because it does not fully control their symptoms. While hot flushes and night sweats usually improve during the first month of treatment, this can take up to three months. Vaginal dryness may take up to six months to improve, and for emotional symptoms such as irritability, anxiety or low mood it may take up to a year to gain the full beneficial effects.

Some women stop because of side-effects. When you first start to take HRT, it is important to know that you will probably notice some short-term changes. Your body has become used to a particular level of oestrogen, and as soon as you start HRT your levels will quickly rise. Your tissues that have become starved of oestrogen are therefore extra sensitive to it and you may notice effects such as breast tenderness, sensitive nipples, leg cramps, mild headaches, mild nausea or discomfort in the stomach area. These effects are common and are likely to be worse in women who have previously experienced prolonged breast tenderness or severe nausea during pregnancy (which suggests they are more sensitive to these effects of oestrogen). The symptoms are not side-effects as such, but the natural response your body makes to oestrogen replenishment, and they are temporary – they usually disappear within one or two cycles. If they last more than three cycles, you may need your dose of oestrogen reduced. There is a small increased risk of deep vein thrombosis (DVT) in the first six months of treatment, but most side-effects associated with HRT are mild and improve over the first three to four months of treatment. If you do experience troublesome side-effects, it is usually possible to reduce the hormone dose you are taking, to switch to a different blend of hormones, or to a different type of HRT (e.g. patches, or skin gel rather than tablets).

Despite the common worry that HRT will make you put on weight, there is no evidence of this. In fact, in one study, more women who were not taking HRT gained weight than those who were taking it.

HRT and Breast Cancer

A common reason for stopping HRT is fear of breast cancer, although the overall increase in risk is thought to be low. It is generally accepted that around 45 out of every 1,000 women aged 50 years who are *not* taking HRT will be diagnosed as having breast cancer before the age of 70 years. In those using HRT for five years, this figures rises by two extra cases per 1,000 women, in those using HRT for ten years it rises by six extra cases per 1,000 women. The benefits of taking HRT are believed to outweigh this small increased risk, as breast cancers developing in women using HRT are less likely to spread beyond the breast than in women not using HRT. As with all women, however, it is important to be breast aware and to accept offers for regular screening mammograms. Once you have obtained the long-term benefits of HRT and you and your doctor decide it is time to stop taking it, the small increased risk of breast cancer disappears within five years of stopping.

One recent trial found that of over 1,000 women aged 50–64 who had taken HRT for eight years, there was no overall association between risk of breast cancer and having taken HRT. Other research found that among women who had taken HRT for at least 15 years following previous breast cancer therapy, there was no increased risk of a recurrence of disease even in those whose tumours were oestrogen sensitive. This suggests that, as many doctors now believe, a history of breast cancer is no longer an absolute contraindication to taking HRT for its other health benefits in the future. However, a recent well-publicized trial did find a higher risk of breast cancer with one particular blend of oestrogen and progestogen (not available in the UK) and as a result further research is needed to help clarify exactly what the risks are (see page 267) as the issues is currently surrounded by confusion.

The thought of breast cancer is enough to strike fear in any woman's heart. But although the statistics look frightening – one in nine women will develop the disease at some time in their life, with 30,000 new cases diagnosed in England and Wales each year – all is not doom and gloom. According to the charity Cancer Research UK, the five-year survival rate for women diagnosed with breast cancer is now as high as 74 per cent and rising, thanks to earlier diagnosis and the availability of improved treatments.

As 90 per cent of breast lumps are found by women or their partners, aim to be breast aware and to know how your own breasts feel while in the bath, shower or dressing. Some breasts are naturally more lumpy than others but subtle changes can be detected.

One in three women will discover a lump in their breasts at some time during their life – the important thing is not to panic. Nine out of ten breast lumps are benign fibrous lumps (fibroadenomas) or fluid-filled cysts, but all need to be investigated just in case. A simple procedure known as a needle aspiration allows a few cells to be collected from the lump, or you may be advised to have the lump removed under a local or general anaesthetic instead. Cells are then examined under a microscope to detect cancerous changes.

If you are diagnosed with breast cancer, you are likely to have some form of surgery. Your cancer specialist needs to advise whether removal of the lump alone is sufficient, or whether a mastectomy is your best option. The next decision is whether you would then benefit from radiotherapy, chemotherapy and/or an anti-oestrogen drug which encourages hormone-sensitive breast tumours to shrink. These decisions will depend on the size of the tumour, the type of cells it contains, how aggressive they are and what stage your disease has reached (i.e. whether it has started to invade local tissues or spread elsewhere).

For women whose breast cancer is discovered while still small and in the early stages (1 and 2), removal of the lump plus a course of radiotherapy or chemotherapy is usually offered, as this approach appears to be as safe and effective as mastectomy.

Several drugs have recently shown exciting results against breast cancer. The anti-oestrogen drug, tamoxifen, is one of the mainstays of treatment for post-menopausal women with hormone-sensitive breast cancer. A recent study involving 9,366 post-menopausal women compared the use of either tamoxifen or a newer drug, anastrozole. Three-year disease-free survival was found to be 2 per cent greater among women given anastrozole alone (89.4 per cent) compared with those given tamoxifen (87.4 per cent). This has been hailed as the biggest step forward in breast cancer treatment for 20 years.

Recent results from another trial found that women with early-stage breast cancer who received a chemotherapy regime including a drug called docetaxel were 32 per cent less likely to experience a recurrence of their cancer than those receiving other treatments. The most significant benefits were in women who had one to three lymph nodes positive for breast cancer cells, which accounts for two out of three women with node-positive, early-stage breast cancer. In these women, risk of relapse was reduced by 50 per cent.

SELF HELP

To help decrease your risk of breast cancer, it is worth:

- following a low-fat, high-fibre diet – in particular, cut back on your intake of saturated fats
- eating at least five servings of fruit or vegetables per day – these contain antioxidants (e.g. vitamins C, E, carotenoids) and substances that seem to protect against cancer such as isoflavones, limonene, sulphoraphane and ellagic acid
- eating more oily fish – essential fatty acids in fish oils can halt the growth of some cancer cells and reverse weight loss in cancer patients
- losing any excess weight – fatty tissues can make oestrogen hormone from other circulating hormones
- taking regular exercise

- avoiding excess alcohol, which boosts the effects of oestrogen. Some research suggests that just drinking one unit of alcohol per day increases the risk of breast cancer by 11 per cent, two units daily increases it by 24 per cent while three units daily may increase the risk by 38 per cent. Sadly, it does not seem that red wine, for all its antioxidant properties, is protective against breast cancer.

HRT and DVT

There is a small increased risk of developing a blood clot in the deep veins of the legs (deep vein thrombosis) which may break off and travel to the lungs to cause sudden chest pain and breathlessness due to a pulmonary embolism (PE). For healthy women on no medication, around five out of every 100,000 women will develop a DVT for no obvious reason per year. For those who are pregnant, the risk rises to around 60 out of every 100,000 pregnant women. For those taking the oral contraceptive Pill, the risk is around 15 to 30 cases per 100,000 women per year. For women taking HRT, the risk is somewhere between five and 15 per 100,000 per year. The risk therefore seems to be low. But for women with a pre-existing risk factor that might be expected to increase the chance of a DVT, such as a personal or family history of DVT or PE, severe varicose vines, obesity, surgery, trauma or prolonged be rest, the risk of taking HRT may be expected to exceed the benefits, and it is important to fully discuss the pros and cons with your doctor before deciding whether or not to continue with HRT.

Possible Side-Effects of HRT

In most cases, the side-effects of HRT are minor, occur at the start of treatment, and settle down within a few weeks. Mild reactions are sometimes helped by changing the dosage or type of HRT. Some are more troublesome, however, so that treatment has to be stopped. Side-effects are listed belows:

- nausea and vomiting
- breast tenderness and enlargement
- breakthrough bleeding
- headache
- dizziness
- leg cramps or muscle pains
- increase in size of uterine fibroids
- intolerance of contact lenses
- skin reactions
- loss of scalp hair
- increase in body or facial hair
- pre-menstrual syndrome
- weight gain
- increased risk of deep vein thrombosis
- increased risk of breast cancer.

HRT Should not be Taken by Women who:

- are pregnant or breast-feeding
- have had an oestrogen-dependent cancer (e.g. of the breast) unless their doctor agrees – an increasing number of experts now feel that women who have been successfully treated for cancer and have no evidence of a recurrence can take HRT

- have undiagnosed vaginal bleeding
- have active endometriosis
- have active blood clotting disorders
- have severe heart, liver or kidney disease.

HRT is only be used with caution and regular check-ups in women who have a medical history of any of the following conditions:

- migraine
- gall stones
- epilepsy
- diabetes
- high blood pressure
- fibroids of the womb
- a history of blood clotting disorders
- mild ongoing liver disease
- a type of deafness called otosclerosis
- skin itching during pregnancy (pruritis)
- a rare blistering skin disease of pregnancy called herpes gestationis
- multiple sclerosis
- a rare, metabolic disease called porphyria
- tetany.

When to Seek Medical Advice

You should stop treatment and seek immediate medical advice if you are taking HRT and develop:

- a first occurrence of migraine
- frequent, severe headaches
- sudden visual disturbances

- possible signs of a blood clot such as pain and swelling of a limb, poor circulation or discoloration of part of the body
- jaundice
- pregnancy.

While some doctors recommend that HRT is stopped six weeks before major planned surgery, others no longer feel this is necessary for normal, low-dose HRT – as long as heparin, a blood thinning agent, is given after surgery. Seek advice from your doctor for the current opinion in your local hospital.

Selective Estrogen Receptor Modulators (SERMs)

A Selective Estrogen[1] Receptor Modulator is a substance that selectively mimics the effects of oestrogen in some tissues while blocking oestrogen effects (or having little action) in other tissues. One of the most important SERMs currently under investigation for use in the prevention and treatment of osteoporosis is a drug called raloxifene.

Oestrogen receptors in different tissues are subtly different in ways that are not yet fully understood. As a result, compounds that mimic the effect of oestrogen in one tissue (e.g. bone) may have the opposite, or no effect, in another oestrogen-sensitive tissue (e.g. breast).

Substances that mimic the effects of oestrogen are known as oestrogen agonists, while those that oppose its effects are called oestrogen antagonists. Antagonists often work by

[1] American spelling of oestrogen

binding to a receptor and tying it up, so that the substance it normally interacts with (in this case oestrogen) cannot reach it to trigger its usual effects.

A SERM may be both an oestrogen agonist and an oestrogen antagonist, depending on the tissue it is in. For example, raloxifene binds readily to oestrogen receptors in the breast and uterus and prevents human oestrogen from binding, resulting in antagonism and reduced risk of over-stimulation. In bone, however, it binds to the oestrogen receptor and stimulates an oestrogen-like effect to help increase production of healthy bone.

SERMS and Osteoporosis

Bone remodelling takes place in so-called bone modelling units (BMUs). These contain:

- osteoclast cells which break down old bone to form small pits
- scavenger cells which briefly move in to a newly formed pit and lay down a film of cement
- osteoblasts which enter the resorption zone, stick to the cement line and refill the pit with new bone.

Lack of oestrogen such as occurs after the menopause leads to:

- increased numbers of BMUs
- the formation of deeper pits within each BMU
- less active osteoblasts which produce less bone to fill each pit.

As a result, more bone is resorbed and less is laid down, so that bones become thin, brittle and fracture more easily.

Oestrogen receptors have been found in osteoblast cells and also in some cells within the bone marrow. It now seems likely that oestrogen and raloxifene help to prevent osteoporosis through:

- a direct action on osteoblast cells to boost their activity
- an indirect action on primitive osteoblast cells in bone marrow that has beneficial effects on their differentiation and activation
- an effect on calcium metabolism which is not yet fully understood.

Because a SERM can stimulate some oestrogen sensitive tissues without affecting others, it can be targeted to help prevent or treat osteoporosis and, unlike pure oestrogen, can still be used in women who have not had a hysterectomy or with an increased risk of breast cancer, as it does not overstimulate the uterus or breasts.

Unfortunately, raloxifene does not reduce menopausal symptoms of hot flushes and night sweats.

Properties of SERMs compared with those of oestrogen

	Oestrogen	1st Generation SERM	2nd Generation SERM
Example	17β-oestradiol	tamoxifen	raloxifene
Effect on heart disease risk factors	agonist	agonist	agonist
Effect on bone	agonist	agonist	agonist
Effect on uterus	agonist	partial agonist	antagonist
Effect on breasts	agonist	antagonist	antagonist

Agonist: mimics oestrogen effect Antagonist: opposes oestrogen effect

Isoflavones (see page 183) are considered to be possible selective estrogen receptor modulators, but possess non-hormonal properties that also may contribute to their effects.

Natural Progesterone

Natural progesterone is gaining in popularity as a form of hormone replacement therapy. Like many synthetic hormones, natural progesterone is derived from plants such as the wild yam (*Dioscorea villosa*) and soya beans. It is important to know that these creams do not contain extracts of wild yam or soya, however – several chemical changes are made to the steroid precursors found in these plants to synthesize progesterone. It is labelled 'natural' as it has the same chemical structure as the progesterone naturally found in the human body – not because it is a natural extract. Natural progesterone cream is therefore just another form of hormone replacement therapy – in this case, progesterone replacement instead of the usual HRT combination of an oestrogen plus a progestogen.

Natural progesterone cannot be given by mouth as it is quickly broken down in the gut (hence synthetic versions, progestogens, are used for oral HRT). It is therefore given as a suppository or as a topical cream to be absorbed into the circulation across a mucous membrane or the skin. Some research suggests it does not cross the skin into the blood stream very well, however, and tends to accumulate in the underlying fat cells. Nevertheless, some experts believe that progesterone cream has a beneficial effect on bones to increase bone density. In one trial, post-menopausal women showed as much as a 10–25 per cent increase in bone mineral density after 12 months treatment.

It is important to point out that in this trial women were also advised to:

- include green, leafy vegetables in their diet
- exercise three times a week
- reduce consumption of cigarettes, alcohol and red meat
- take supplements of calcium, vitamin D and vitamin C
- some also took oestrogen for three weeks per month if appropriate, although the effect of oestrogen plus progesterone cream was found not to be superior to progesterone cream (plus diet and lifestyle changes) without oestrogen.

The effects of progesterone cream alone are still under investigation, as many women do find it helpful. In one study of 102 women, 83 per cent using progesterone cream for one year reported improvements in hot flushes, compared with only 19 per cent on placebo. Creams containing wild yam extract (diosgenin) itself are also interesting. Recent research suggests extracts help to lower the high levels of FSH and LH hormones associated with menopausal symptoms. A number of fact sheets, including one on progesterone cream, are available from the Natural Menopause Advice Service (see Useful Addresses Addresses for contact details).

Bisphosphonates

Bisphosphonates (e.g. alendronate, risedronate, etidronate) are drugs that help to protect against osteoporosis in menopausal women. They work by blocking the action of cells which break down old bones so that bone-building bones can keep up with them and build more new bone. They have been shown to:

- slow the rate at which bone is resorbed
- stimulate production of new bone
- reduce the risk of bone fracture.

As well as being used to treat established osteoporosis, bisphosphonates are now also used to prevent osteoporosis in women at high risk. Research shows they can build up bones in the spine, wrist and hip to reduce the risk of a fracture by as much as 88 per cent in post-menopausal women.

Etidronate is given in 90-day cycles for two weeks every three months: etidronate for 14 days, followed by effervescent calcium carbonate tablets for 76 days. It is mainly active on the bones in the back, which reduces the risk of vertebral osteoporotic fractures.

Alendronate is considered to be 100 times more powerful than etidronate. It is taken either once a day or, in post-menopausal women once weekly, to strengthen bone at all sites to reduce the risk of spinal, wrist and hip fractures by over 50 per cent. The risk of having two or more spinal fractures is reduced by as much as 90 per cent.

Possible Side-effects

These include:

- abdominal pain and distension
- flatulence
- diarrhoea or constipation
- muscle and bone pain
- headache
- rash

Calcitonin

Calcitonin is a hormone injection, originally derived from salmon but now made synthetically. It helps to regulate bone turn-over and increases bone density in women with osteoporosis. It is used to treat rather than prevent osteoporosis and works by suppressing resorption of calcium from old bone. It is given daily (by nasal spray, or injection), together with calcium and vitamin D supplements.

Possible Side-effects

These include:

- nausea
- vomiting
- diarrhoea
- flushing
- dizziness
- tingling of hands
- unpleasant taste
- abdominal pain
- local irritation at delivery site.

14
Sexuality and the Menopause

Falling levels of oestrogen as the menopause approaches affects fertility, your contraceptive needs and your sexuality.

Fertility

A woman in her late forties or early fifties who is approaching the menopause is less than half as fertile as a woman in her twenties, but can still become pregnant. Although the menopause signals the end of your fertile life, many women continue to produce small surges of oestrogen. These may be enough to trigger the occasional release of an egg. Many pregnancies occurring over the age of 40 are unplanned. Unless a woman would like to have a child at this time of life, it is important to use an effective method of contraception, as pregnancy in older women does carry additional health risks:

- the maternal mortality rate in the age group 40–49 is four times higher than for pregnant women aged 20–29
- the risk of a perinatal death for the baby is doubled as maternal age doubles
- chromosome abnormalities in the fetus (e.g. Down's syndrome) are increasingly likely over the age of 35.

Contraception

If you do not wish to become pregnant, you need to use a reliable method of contraception for at least one year after your last period – as long as this takes you over the age of 50. If you are still under 50, you should used contraception for a total of two years after your last period. The options available include:

- natural fertility awareness
- Persona
- male condom
- female condom
- diaphragm
- coil (IUCD)
- intra-uterine system (progestogen coil called Mirena)
- mini (progestogen only) – Pill
- combined oral contraceptive Pill
- depot progestogen injection
- progestogen implants.

Your pharmacist, practice nurse or doctor can advise on which method is likely to suit you best.

Sexual Relationships

Many women find that sex feels different after the menopause as a result of falling oestrogen levels. This can have both psychological and physical effects on your sex life. Not surprisingly, symptoms can lead to relationship difficulties and many women become depressed. In most cases, you will start to feel better as your body gets used to lower levels of oestrogen hormone. It can be difficult for your sexual partner to understand what you are going through at this time of life, however. The important thing is to communicate – don't be afraid to let your partner know how you are feeling.

A rewarding sex life is an important part of well-being and a loving relationship, yet many couples come face to face with sexual problems in later life. Often, these problems are accepted with resignation, yet loss of sexuality should not be viewed as an inevitable part of the ageing process – it is not. A recent survey of over 1,300 older people by the National Council on Aging (NCA) in the US found that nearly 60 per cent of men and women over the age of 60 were still fully sexually active.

The majority did report having sex less often than when they were younger, however, and around 40 per cent felt they would like to have sex more often than they did. More than one in three men in their sixties and half of men in their seventies also admitted they had been unable to consistently obtain and maintain an erection during the previous six months, while one in three women found that lack of lubrication could be a problem.

Sexual problems do become more frequent as you get older, especially in women who have had a natural menopause or who have had their ovaries and uterus removed (bilateral oophorectomy and total hysterectomy).

Types of FSD (Female Sexual Dysfunction) that have been associated with the menopause include:

- delayed sexual arousal
- vaginal dryness
- pain on intercourse (dyspareunia)
- painful orgasm
- delayed orgasm or lack of orgasm (anorgasmia)
- urinary symptoms after intercourse
- reduced sexual drive
- lack of sensitivity in the clitoris
- over-sensitivity of the clitoris
- generalized changes in skin touch sensations which may make skin contact feel unpleasant.

An anonymous survey of female patients registered with four doctors' surgeries found that 41 per cent admitted to having a current sexual problem. Of these, the most common types of FSD were vaginal dryness (28 per cent), difficulty obtaining orgasm (27 per cent), painful intercourse (18 per cent), inhibited enjoyment (18 per cent) and problems with arousal (17 per cent). A similar survey in the US found that 32 per cent of women reported low or no sexual desire. This contributed to other sexual difficulties including vaginal dryness (21 per cent) and painful sexual intercourse (16 per cent). Overall, almost one in four women (23 per cent) in this study no longer found sex pleasurable.

Frequency of sexual activity varies from couple to couple at this time of life. Out of 182 women aged 48 to 58 years, 18 per cent of women were sexually active several times per week, 48 per cent once a week, 27 per cent less than once a week and 7 per cent were not sexually active at all.

Unfortunately, FSD can mean that older women are less

likely to remain sexually active. One study involving 448 women aged 60 or over found that only 56 per cent of those who were married were still sexually active. There was also a significant decrease in sexual activity with increasing age.

Hormone changes occurring as a result of the menopause are frequently to blame. When 39 women were followed from around the time of the menopause until one year after their last menstrual cycle, researchers found that while all the women were sexually active at the start of the study, only around 50 per cent were still sexual active by the end of the study. A large review of 16 studies of female sexuality after the menopause found that women experience a consistent decrease in sexual interest, frequency of sexual activity, frequency of orgasms and in lubrication after the menopause.

Vaginal Dryness

The most noticeable physical effect of lack of oestrogen is vaginal dryness. Every woman will notice this to some extent after the menopause unless you are taking HRT. Lack of lubrication means it is more difficult to become aroused and sex may be painful due to dryness. The clitoris also becomes less sensitive. In most cases, using a special water-based lubricant gel or pessaries will help to revitalize a flagging sex life.

If the problem continues, it is important to see your doctor. There is a condition called Sjögren's Syndrome in which the eyes, mouth, nose, throat or vagina can start to dry up. This is linked with the immune system attacking the normal lubricating glands. Nine out of ten sufferers are women, mostly over the age of 30. If you have also noticed dry, gritty eyes, this condition is a possibility. It is not particularly serious, but you will probably need treatment with lubricants such as artificial tears or saliva.

Clitoral Hood Retraction

After the menopause, the tissues around your vagina naturally shrink and thin down due to lack of oestrogen. In some women, the hood covering the clitoris becomes retracted. This exposes sensitive tissues full of nerve endings that may make sexual stimulation intensely unpleasant. If this happens, don't be afraid to confide in your doctor. Oestrogen replacement, either locally with cream or vaginal tablets will quickly solve the problem.

Loss of Skin Sensitivity

Unfortunately for women, the skin all over your body becomes less sensitive as oestrogen levels fall. One study found that six out of ten post-menopausal women noticed skin numbness, so that caresses from their partner were no longer enjoyable. Not surprisingly, nine out of ten of these women found this sensory loss interfered with their enjoyment of sex.

You may find that your skin sensitivity improves if your partner gives you a sensual massage. Use a ready-made sensual massage lotion or make one yourself by diluting one or more essential oils in a carrier such as sweet almond oil – use 15–30 drops essential oils per 30 ml carrier oil. Aromatherapy essential oils that have sensual properties include:

- ylang ylang
- tuberose

- jasmine
- rose otto
- rose maroc
- sandalwood.

You may also find that taking an Evening Primrose Oil supplement and following a diet rich in plant hormones helps. In most cases, HRT will quickly bring skin sensitivity back up to normal.

Difficulty Reaching Orgasm

One in six menopausal women find it more and more difficult to reach orgasm. This is probably due to lowered sensitivity of the clitoris as oestrogen levels fall.

Normally, during female sexual arousal, fluid is secreted into the vagina to provide lubrication. The upper third of the vagina lengthens and expands, becoming very sensitive to touch. The entrance to the vagina becomes swollen and tighter to grip the penis more firmly. During orgasm, nerve impulses spread through various nerves to cause contraction of pelvic floor muscles and sometimes your thigh muscles as well.

When oestrogen levels are low, however, vaginal lubrication is scant. Because your vaginal tissues are also starting to shrink, expansion of the upper vagina and tightening of the lower vagina may not occur. There are also changes in the way your nerves conduct electrical impulses, which mean that orgasm is more difficult to achieve and when it does occur, sensation is less intense – this is also linked to weakening of pelvic floor muscles and stress incontinence.

A study in which ultrasound probes recorded what happened during intercourse in women found that when the male penetrated a woman from behind or the side, she achieved a better orgasm than in the Missionary position, and it is worth trying different positions until you find one that suits you best.

Loss of Sex Drive

Loss of sex drive is the commonest sexual problem to affect women, especially after the menopause. Your sex drive is controlled by the interaction of the female hormones, oestrogen and progesterone plus the male hormone, testosterone. The level of testosterone in women is much lower than that in men and varies widely. Women who have higher levels of active testosterone tend to have a higher sex drive. Testosterone in women is mainly produced by the ovaries, so after the menopause, testosterone levels usually fall, although small amounts of testosterone-like hormones (androgens) are also made by:

- the adrenal glands
- the skin
- muscle cells
- the brain and pineal gland
- hair follicles
- body fat stores.

During the menopause, these other androgen sources take over testosterone production from the ovaries and their output of androgen hormones doubles. In some women, this is so successful that your sex drive may even increase as testosterone effects become more pronounced without oestrogen to counter-balance them.

Although it is difficult to talk about embarrassing

problems such as a falling sex drive, it is important to talk to your partner and find out how they feel. Any frequency of making love is normal so long as both of you are happy about it. Many couples share love, affection and a meaningful emotional relationship without a physically active sex life. Frequently, however, particularly where making love has virtually petered out, one of the partners will be unhappy about the lack of a physical relationship. Over a third of menopausal women feel that men want sex more often than they do themselves.

Loss of sex drive may not necessarily be due to the menopause. It is natural for sexual activity to decline the longer you have been in a relationship. You may need to work out why your desires have changed.

- Are there other problems in your relationship?
- Do you find time to talk?
- Are you too tied up with work, running the home or caring for relatives?
- Do you are your partner still show affection for each other?
- Are you still friends?

If you still show affection towards each other and you still enjoy a cuddle together, lack of sex drive is unlikely to be due to one or other of you falling out of love, or to problems in your relationship. It may well be linked to your changing hormones, although it can also be linked with tiredness, anxiety, stress or illness. The following suggestions may help.

1. Make sure you get plenty of sleep – tiredness will quickly lower your libido.

2. Avoid excessive stress – take regular time out for rest and relaxation.

3. Take more exercise – this will boost your metabolic rate, improve your fitness level and burn off excess stress hormones – don't overdo it, however.

4. If you smoke, try to stop – research shows that smoking lowers hormone levels enough to bring the menopause on up to two years earlier than normal and also affects your sex drive.

5. Avoid drinking excessive amounts of alcohol. In the long term, this can lower your sex drive, reduce vaginal secretions, shrink the ovaries and lead to menstrual problems. The intakes that trigger these problems vary from person to person, depending on how your metabolism handles alcohol and how much exercise you take. Stick to no more than 2 to 3 units per day for women.

6. Take a good multinutrient supplement – lack of some vitamins and minerals, especially zinc, can cause hormonal imbalances and reduce your sex drive.

7. Try also taking Evening Primrose Oil supplements – these contain essential fatty acids that act as building blocks for sex hormones.

8. Check that a low sex drive is not an unwanted side-effect of any tablets you are taking – those that can affect your libido include drugs prescribed for high blood pressure, water retention and depression.

Studies show that women gain significant quality of sex life benefits from HRT including: increased sexual frequency and enjoyment sexual fantasies and vaginal lubrication, and decreased pain during intercourse.

Hysterectomy and Your Sex Drive

If your menopause has come on following a hysterectomy, you are more likely to notice changes in your sex life. When making love, the uterus moves upwards as you become aroused. During orgasm, it contracts rhythmically to add to the intense sensations felt during climax. One in three women who have had a hysterectomy notice the loss of these uterine sensations when making love and seven out of ten find it more difficult to achieve orgasm. Although there may be no difference in your sex drive at first, after a year women who have had a hysterectomy have significantly fewer orgasms per year than women with an intact womb. In a few cases, the opposite is true – some women find love-making more enjoyable and orgasm more intense after the operation, especially if they were previously in a lot of pain.

Painful Sex

Deep pain during intercourse may be due to diseased ovaries, a prolapsed womb, or to the bladder or rectum bulging into the vagina to form a cystocoele or rectocoele. These problems often develop after the menopause as lack of oestrogen allows pelvic tissues to thin and stretch.

If intercourse suddenly becomes painful for no obvious reason, it is important to tell your doctor. Both superficial and deep pain during intercourse have a variety of causes, including a thrush infection, bacterial imbalance, endometriosis, an ovarian cyst or even an ectopic pregnancy. In most cases, the problem can be solved with proper investigation and treatment.

Seeking Help

If you have a sex problem that seems to be related to the menopause, it is best to seek help from your GP. If you have a physical problem such as vaginal dryness or painful intercourse, this needs to be investigated to make sure there is no infection or other problem present. Treatment with vaginal lubricants or HRT will often help to sort the situation out.

If you feel the sexual problem is linked to your relationship rather than the menopause, contact Relate. Their local number will be in the telephone directory. Relate have a number of counsellors and sex therapists who are trained to help anyone cope with a relationship or sexual problem – sympathetically and in confidence.

Loss of sex drive that is not linked with other signs of oestrogen withdrawal such as thinning of vagina tissues may improve with combined oestrogen and testosterone therapy. Testosterone is a male hormone and is only usually prescribed to women by a doctor specializing in the area of menopausal problems.

Sensate Focusing

Sex therapists sometimes advise a form of treatment known as sensate focusing, or pleasuring, to help overcome lack of interest in sex. At first, penetrative sex is banned and a couple takes turns to caress and explore each others body during foreplay. You are encouraged to spend around an hour giving each other pleasure through massage, but avoiding obviously erotic areas such as the breasts and genitals. Once both partners are comfortable with this, you progress to the next stage of Genital Sensate Focusing, in which erogenous zones can be touched as well.

Mutual masturbation is allowed, but full intercourse remains out of bounds. This takes away any pressure to perform and allows the woman to relax without fearing intercourse. Eventually, sometimes after more than 20 sessions lasting an hour each, simple vaginal penetration without subsequent thrusting may be achieved. Later, penile thrusting is introduced as well.

Sex Positions to Try

Women-on-top positions help you to gain better control during love-making and can prove more satisfying for both of you. By moving up and down and varying the speed and depth of penetration, you can set your own pace so you are likely to reach orgasm more easily. These positions are also good if you are particularly tired.

FOR BETTER CONTROL: UPSIDE-DOWN MISSIONARY POSITION
With your partner lying on his back and you lying on top, gently guide his penis into you. Bring your legs inside his to increase the friction between his penis and your vagina and clitoris.

FOR BETTER AROUSAL: OPEN ACCESS POSITION
With your partner lying on his back, sit on top of him and lean back, balancing yourself by resting both hands on his knees or thighs. Your partner can then reach forward to caress and massage your breasts or gently stimulate your clitoris as you move up and down.

FOR A MORE INTENSE ORGASM: PENETRATION FROM BEHIND

Sexual penetration from behind can give you a more satisfying orgasm as this thins and stretches the front wall of the vagina where the mystical G-spot is said to be situated. Lean forward from the hips, either while standing up or when kneeling on a bed or armchair. Support yourself by holding onto the bedhead or back of the chair. Your partner should penetrate you gently from behind while holding onto your waist or buttocks. This lets him achieve deep penetration. Another position good for stimulating the G-spot is to make love when lying curled up, side by side, with his front to your back (Spoons Position).

Treatment

If you experience sexual difficulties, don't be embarrassed to discuss these with your doctor. Female sexual problems can usually be readily overcome with one of the many medical treatments now available. Often simple remedies such as using a water-based lubricating gel can help. HRT (e.g. oestrogen cream containing 0.1 per cent estradiol) or a vaginal gel based on natural isoflavones can have a beneficial effect. An oral isoflavone supplement will also help.

One of the factors that has been associated with decreased female sexual activity after the menopause is a decline in testosterone levels. Even though testosterone is often referred to as the male sex hormone, women produce small amounts in their ovaries and in outer layer of their adrenal glands (the cortex). Blood levels of testosterone are around 18 times lower in women than in men, however.

Although variations in testosterone level within the normal range may not affect female sexual function significantly, women with a higher testosterone level may experience increased desire compared with women with lower testosterone levels. After the menopause, both oestrogen and testosterone levels start to fall. Testosterone levels are more likely to be associated with both frequency of female sexual desire and with the level of sexual activity. As a result, some experts have suggested that low, 'non-masculinizing' doses of testosterone might help women with FSD as a result of hormonal changes occurring after a natural menopause or after surgical removal of the uterus and ovaries.

Complementary Treatments that can help

HERBALISM

Catuaba promotes erotic dreams in both men and women, followed by increased sexual desire within 5–21 days of regular treatment. Damiana produces localized tingling and throbbing sensations in the genitals and increases sensitivity of nerve endings. Muira Puama stimulates desire through a direct action on brain chemicals, stimulating nerve endings in the genitals and by promoting the effects of testosterone. Korean and American Ginseng can help the body adapt to physical and emotional stress and are widely reputed to have an aphrodisiac effect. Siberian Ginseng is also noted for its aphrodisiac properties. In post-menopausal women, St John's Wort helps 60 per cent become interested in sex again after three months of treatment. *Tribulus terrestris* – a plant widely used in Indian Ayurvedic medicine – is now also available and works by increasing the effects of testosterone, especially where reduced activity is associated with stress, tiredness and fatigue.

HOMEOPATHY

Homeopathic hormones such as testosterone or oestrogen are used by some practitioners to normalize hormone imbalances associated with loss of libido, especially in those unable to take orthodox hormone replacement therapy. The following specific remedies are taken at 6 c potency twice a day for up to a week:

- for low sex drive linked with lethargy, stress or feelings of guilt about sex: *Phosphoricum acidum*
- for low sex drive linked with anxiety and fear of failure: *Arsenicum album*
- for low sex drive linked with physical exhaustion and mental fatigue: *Cuprum metallicum*
- for low sex drive linked with anxiety, depression and other strong emotions, especially those that are suppressed: *Natrum muriaticum*
- for low sex drive in those who are workaholic, stressed, irritable, over-active, have difficulty sleeping and indulge in excess alcohol, caffeine or cigarettes: *Nux vomica*
- for low sex drive linked with listlessness, lethargy, sluggishness and stress: *Phosphoricum acidum*.

AROMATHERAPY

The heavy, floral essential oils of geranium, rose, jasmine and ylang ylang are among the most powerful aromatic aphrodisiacs. Other essential oils that can increase sex drive include black pepper, cardamom, cinnamon (for perfuming air only – do not bring into contact with the skin) and ginger.

Useful Addresses

Women's Nutritional Advisory Service
PO Box 268,
Lewes
Sussex BN7 2QN
Tel.: 01273 487366
www.wnas.org.uk
Advice and nutritional information for treating menopausal
symptoms and osteoporosis (a fee is payable).

Natural Menopause Advice Service
NMAS, PO Box 71
Leatherhead
Surrey
KT22 7DP
FREEPHONE 0800 1692163
www.nmas.org.uk

National Osteoporosis Society
Camerton
Bath
BA2 0PJ
Helpline: 01761 472721
www.nos.org.uk

British Heart Foundation
14 Fitzhardinge Street
London
W1H 4DH
Tel.: 0207 935 0185
www.bhf.org.uk

QUIT
211 Old Street
London
EC1V 9NR
Smokers' Quitline: 0800 002200
www.quit.org.uk
Advice and counselling on giving up smoking.

Relate
Herbert Gray College
Little Church Street
Rugby
Warwickshire
CV21 3AP
Tel.: 01788 573241
www.relate.org.uk

The British Acupuncture Council
63 Jeddo Road
London
W12 9HQ
Tel.: 020 8735 0400
www.acupuncture.org.uk

The British Medical Acupuncture Society
12 Marbury House
Higher Whitley
Warrington
Cheshire
WA4 4JA
Tel.: 01925 730727
www.medical-acupuncture.co.uk

General Chiropractic Council
344–354 Gray's Inn Road
LONDON
WC1X 8BP
United Kingdom
Tel: 020 7713 5155
www.gcc-uk.org

The International Register of Consultant Herbalists and Homeopaths
32 King Edward Road
Swansea
SA1 4LL
Tel.: 01792 655 886
www.irch.org

National Institute of Medical Herbalists
56 Longbrooke Street
Exeter
EX4 6AH
Tel.: 01392 426022
www.nimh.org.uk

European Herbal Practitioners Association
45A Corsica Street
London
N5 1JT
Tel.: 020 7354 5067
www.users.globalnet.co.uk/~ehpa

British Homeopathic Association
15 Clerkenwell Close
London
EC1R 0AA
Tel.: 020 7566 7800
www.trusthomeopathy.org

General Osteopathic Council
Osteopathy House
176 Tower Bridge Road
London
SE1 3LU
Tel.:0207 357 6655, ext 242
www.osteopathy.org.uk

Index